DOMINATE

Conquer your fears. Become the man you want to be.

David De Las Morenas

ISBN-13: 978-1497518162

ISBN-10: 1497518164

BUYER BONUS

Thank you for buying *Dominate.* Visit **www.HowToBeast.com/Masculinity-Mistakes** to download *Masculinity Mistakes* for free. This eBook details seven commons mistakes men make that limit their confidence and success.

CONTENTS

INTRODUCTION: ESCAPING THE AGE OF WEAKNESS

Look around you.

What do you see?

Do you see great men conquering their fears and living a life they enjoy – a life that they chose? Or are they living a life that was chosen for them?

More importantly, are you living a life that you consciously decided on – one that you handpicked based on your personal preferences and desires?

Unfortunately for most men in today's world, the answer is a loud and resounding **no**. The average man has been following the path of least resistance since he was born.

His childhood and adolescence were the highlights of his life. By the time he's entered the labor market and reached 30, he's all but given up on seeking out new life experiences. Instead of looking for continued growth or further accomplishment, he's living in a state of contempt and resentment.

He spends the majority of his time working in a cubicle that he despises, because it was the first or only job offered to him. He dates or marries a girl that he's barely even attracted to, because she was a friend of a friend and practically fell into his lap. Or he's lonely and single.

Yes, there's a small subset of men who live a life they thoroughly enjoy – one that they've intentionally created. They work for themselves or at a job they deliberately selected, and they date several girls at once, or just one that they're authentically attracted to and who adds measurable value to their life.

But these men are the exception. They only constitute a fraction of a percentage of the population.

The average modern man is on the decline. He's moving farther and farther away being the independent and confident adventurer, and closer and closer to being the social recluse, content with his average life.

Gentlemen, welcome to the age of weakness, where standing out and seeking what you want is not only rare, but also looked down upon by the jealous masses.

They hate to see someone break free from the chains that have held them captive, stopping them from making positive changes or seeking a life that they truly want – especially if it's a friend or close acquaintance. It only serves to remind them of their own fears and insecurities – the ones that they don't have the balls to confront.

At this point, I must stop and ask you the following questions:

Will you be held back? Will you let the increasingly average lifestyle of the day be forced upon you?

Or will you break free and actually work towards creating a life that you want? Will you cease to be another mindless freak that simply lives and reacts?

I hope you answered no to the first two questions and yes to the second two. Otherwise the contents of this book will fall upon deaf ears.

The only way to break free from this self-devouring cycle is **aggressively**.

You must consciously and forcefully dominate life until you find a way out – better yet, until you ***create*** *a way out.*

You can't wait for the right moment. You can't wait for the

perfect set of circumstances. You can't wait for someone else's hand to pull you out, either. You're born alone and you die alone. At the end of the day you're the only person you can count on.

It's up to you to become a man who dominates life. Otherwise, you're destined for the default path: being dominated by life. And the symptoms of each of these conditions go far beyond the two examples of work and women that I mentioned above.

For example, the dominant man has a social presence about him that can't be ignored. His aggressive approach to knowing – and getting – what he wants manifests itself in a supreme sense of confidence. He stands tall, smiles, looks you in the eye, and tells you what he must – without a second thought about it.

The average Joe tends to come off as nervous or stand-offish. This is a result of the many underlying insecurities he constantly carries around with him. He's unsure of what he wants, and this puts him in a state of constant fear.

In this book, I'll share an actionable strategy to assist you in dominating life and getting what you want. The book is divided into six parts – the six different aspects of life you must dominate. Each part includes a handful of rules you should follow in order to fully dominate that particular area.

In addition to a set of actionable steps that follow each rule, I've included a large number of historical examples and personal anecdotes throughout. This is so that everything is clearly illustrated and defined.

In my opinion, there's nothing worse than a book full of vague advice and philosophical ramblings. I've gone to lengths to avoid this trap and produce a book that's both practical and useful.

HOW TO READ AND USE THIS BOOK

This book consists of 19 chapters, divided into 6 sections. Each chapter represents a particular rule that should be followed on the path to domination. Each rule contains a set of actionable steps that should be carried out in order to adhere to the rule.

Some of these steps can be implemented immediately, others cannot. Rather, they set a particular direction for you to work towards, or govern how you should react under a certain set of circumstances as you live your life.

For these reasons, I suggest reading through the book and taking notes on the rules that apply most to you – the ones that you're not doing a good job of following at this point in your life.

This includes things that you used to do well, or habits you used to have. Too many people get stuck in the past and refuse to accept or change something, because it didn't used to be an issue.

For each rule, stop and ask yourself: is this something I currently do or adhere to by default? If not, then take note of how or what you need to change going forward to fix this.

After one complete read-through of the book, it makes sense to go through a second time with a more focused approach. You'll know which areas pertain to you most, and you can better concentrate on applying the advice to your own life as a result.

PART I: DEATH

No one can confidently say that he will still be living tomorrow.

- Euripides: ancient Greek writer, 4th century BC

CHAPTER 1

Death plays a central role in Tibetan Buddhist traditions, where it's a frequent focus for their meditations. These meditations often occur at burial grounds or even in the presence of dead and decaying bodies. I don't know of another culture that's so acutely aware of the inevitability of death, and what it means for the living.

This contrasts starkly with modern western cultures that play the dangerous game of ignoring death. We talk about the dead as if they were still alive. We cultivate an environment where talking about death is seen in a negative light. We watch films like *Indiana Jones* and fantasize about elixirs of never-ending life. When one of our own dies, we dress them up in fancy clothes and make-up so that we can see them, and even talk to them as if they were still living.

Nearly everything we do surrounding death is based on the premise of trying to avoid a basic reality: **everyone dies**. The reason we do this is obvious: we like being alive and can't quite fathom the existence of an earth that no longer includes us at its center.

But we can't avoid it. No one has. Not even Jesus. Not even Mohammed. Not even Buddha.

And that brings us back to Tibetan Buddhism, and their strong connection to death. This connection is so important to them because it reminds them that all things are impermanent, even our own existence.

Nowhere is this more obvious than in their *Nine-Point Mediation on Death.* Using this mediation, a practitioner contemplates the following set of truths:

Truth 1: Death is certain

1. We cannot escape death

2. Each moment we're alive brings us one step closer to death

3. Death comes in a single instant and is unexpected

Conclusion: Practice the Dharma (the Buddhist teachings)

Truth 2: The time of death is uncertain

4. The duration of our lives is unpredictable

5. There are more causes for death than causes for life

6. The human body is extremely fragile

Conclusion: Practice the Dharma now

Truth 3: The only thing that can help you at the time of death is your mental and spiritual development

7. Wealth we've accumulated can't help

8. Friends and family can't help

9. Our bodies can't help

Conclusion: Practice the Dharma purely

The Tibetan Buddhists remind themselves of these truths to encourage practice of the Dharma, and to make two important realizations:

1. Recognizing how short and precious life is – with this knowledge they're more likely to make it meaningful and live it fully.

2. Familiarizing themselves with the reality of death – with this knowledge they can remove their fears that stem from the prospect of dying.

Rule 1: Acknowledge your coming death

Death is the most common fear. It's the one destiny that everyone on this planet shares. But in order to dominate life, you must accept the inevitability of death – the inevitability that one day you won't be here.

I'm going to die. You're going to die. Everyone we know is going to die, too.

But if you live in constant fear of death, you're unlikely to have a meaningful or impactful life. You'll spend all of your time worrying about it or shying away from new opportunities because you're afraid of it.

And maybe this cautious attitude will prolong your life by a fraction of a percentage, but at what cost? Reduced productivity, reduced achievement, reduced enjoyment of life – to name a few. Only when you fully accept your morbid fate can you fully embrace and dominate the little time that you do have.

It sounds cliché, but we're all born and we all die. The time in between those events is what defines us. What we do defines who we are. But if we're living in constant denial of the known end to our story, we won't proceed in an authentic way that keeps our best interests in mind.

The truth is that the average modern man exhibits this fear to such a large degree that it paralyzes him. It stops him from doing anything bold. He's so afraid of dying that he barely even lives. When you accept your fate, you separate yourself from the hordes of John Does who can't do the same. You begin to live life on a higher plane of existence.

You must rid yourself of any delusions that you have and accept your own coming death. Only then will you be able to take maximum control and dominate the little time that you do have.

My Experience

Just last week, I was on my laptop at the gym, plugging some new items into my calendar.

"David," I hear a deep voice call out from behind me.

I turn around and see my friend Ned walking towards me. Ned is a big guy, coming in around 6'5" and 250 lbs. "What's up Ned? I thought you were in Panama..."

"I was. Lee passed away," he says, looking down at his Timberland boots.

I'd seen Lee and Ned just days ago at the gym. Lee was only in his 40s. On top of that, he was extremely fit. They were excited, talking about their upcoming trip to Panama. "Oh my god!" I shout, "What happened!? I'm so sorry to hear that."

Ned looks around, searching for words. "The doctors aren't sure. In the middle of the night he started coughing up blood. I didn't know what was going on. I screamed for help. By the time we got to the hospital he was gone. They revived him three times. But they couldn't keep him with us."

All of a sudden, I feel the impulse to cry. I'm friendly with Ned, but barely knew Lee. We always exchanged hellos, but that was about it. I'm shocked that someone in seemingly perfect health can die without a moment's notice. One breath he was here, the next he was gone.

We all know death is a reality, but for the most part, it comes when expected. A grandparent passes away after struggling against Alzheimer's for several years. A soldier dies in the line of duty.

Yes, it's always painful to lose someone, but when it happens unexpectedly it hits that much harder. Why? Because it could have been you. It could have been me.

This recent experience had a large impact on me. I could see the disbelief, shock, and confusion in my friend Ned's eyes as he struggled to piece together words and sentences. It was so real.

Death is so real.

Take Action

The advantages of acknowledging your own coming death are numerous. In a broad sense, it will ground your life in reality, allowing you to approach everything from a more effective, more fearless mindset.

The best way to condition yourself to accept this fact, and live like it, is through frequent reminder. And I don't know of a better reminder than *The Nine-Point Meditation on Death.*

Read the following truths one-by-one, think of any relatable experiences you've had (e.g. people you know who've died). Make it real. Think about your own coming death. This will light a fire under your belly to value what time you do have.

Note: I've altered the conclusions to apply more generally.

Truth 1: Death is certain

1. We cannot escape death

2. Each moment we're alive brings us one step closer to death

3. Death comes in a single instant and is unexpected

Conclusion: Practice things that facilitate personal growth and bring you happiness

Truth 2: The time of death is uncertain

4. The duration of our lives is unpredictable

5. There are more causes for death than causes for life

6. The human body is extremely fragile

Conclusion: Practice things that facilitate personal growth (do it now)

Truth 3: The only thing that can help you at the time of death is your mental and spiritual development

7. Wealth we've accumulated can't help

8. Friends and family can't help

9. Our bodies can't help

Conclusion: Practice things that facilitate personal growth without getting distracted by attachments to material objects or other people

CHAPTER 2

Very few men have been affected by death as much as professional basketball player Stephen Jackson. Growing up in the crime-ridden country city of Port Arthur, Texas, Jackson experienced more than his fair share of death.

One incident came early in his youth. It was 2 or 3 in the morning and Jackson was hanging out with some friends at his buddy Neil's house. He'd snuck out of his own home earlier that night, avoiding his mother's curfew.

While the friends were in the midst of a game of dice, a car full of men from the other side of town drove by and proceeded to fire 48 gunshots towards the house. They had beef with someone at the dice game.

Jackson clearly recalls the trauma. "There was like 9 of us outside, but I didn't get hit. Thank god." Two of his friends weren't so lucky.

If this incident didn't imprint the reality of death on Jackson's mind, a tragedy involving his brother definitely did. Donald Buckner was Jackson's older brother. They shared the same father, but different mothers. Growing up they were inseparable. Jackson shared his first drink with Buckner, who taught him other brotherly things like how to dress and how to talk to girls.

One night, 25 year old Buckner was hanging out at his girlfriend's place. There was a knock at the door. The girlfriend went to answer. It was her ex-boyfriend. She refused to let him in, and told him to get lost.

Later that night when Buckner left the house, the ex was still outside, patiently waiting. He confronted Buckner. The altercation quickly escalated into a fist fight. Just when it looked like Buckner was about to emerge victorious, two men came up from behind him. They beat his head in with a bottle and a lead pipe.

Jackson, then 16, came to visit his brother in the ICU at the hospital hours later, where he was resting in critical condition. 17 staples held his head together. Jackson clasped his brother's hand and told him, "It's all right. We're going to take care of you." Minutes later, Buckner passed. Feeling overwhelmed and completely helpless, Jackson sat there and watched his brother die.

"It's tough, because you never know when it's your turn," Jackson says, looking back on that day. This realization is what inspired him to take his basketball game to the next level, and eventually win an NBA championship with the San Antonio Spurs in 2003.

All of the death he saw gave his life a whole new meaning – a whole new value.

Rule 2: Value your time above all

Once you acknowledge the fact that you're going to die, you must use it as motivation to conquer and accomplish.

Avoid the trap of letting thoughts of your death drain your energy and lower your mood. The time you have on this earth, however short or long it may be, is going to pass regardless of what you do. So you might as well dominate life and leave your imprint where you can.

Conversely, I won't repeat the age-old logic that you should *live everyday like it's your last.* If you were truly to take this to heart, you'd never get anything of real value done, but rather indulge in day-to-day leisurely activities of no lasting value.

The best way you can resolve the conflict of your coming death is to value your time above all. You only have a finite amount of time, so it's of the utmost importance that you use it wisely.

This doesn't mean you have to be a 24/7 productivity machine. Yes, if you want to dominate life and accomplish large goals you must spend the majority of your time working with a conscious focus. But it's equally important to value your down-time.

Don't make the mistake of letting time waste away while you mindlessly browse the internet. Instead, you should decide that you're going to take some time off, and put it towards thoroughly relaxing and taking a vacation or watching and enjoying the story of a book or a movie. Or you can put that downtime towards trying out a new hobby or learning a new skill.

The important thing is to not just let time pass by. There are unlimited ways you can spend your time, just be sure you're doing so in a way that reflects its true value – **the value of your life.**

Stephen Jackson realized this value as he saw the lives of his peers and family members vanish before his very eyes. Instead of letting the prospect of his own death weigh him down into a mind-numbing life of drugs and crime, like most people in his environment, he resolved to use whatever time he had left to dominate the game of basketball and see how far he could go.

You must do as Jackson did. You must value your time on earth more than any material possession – more than any other person. Don't fall for the common trap of wasting your time away watching television and sports like the majority of the mediocre masses. Realize that your time is all you have, and that it's decreasing by the minute. You must use it wisely.

My Experience

In addition to recognizing my coming death, my outlook on why I must value my time above all other things comes as a result of my economics degree.

Arguably the most important economic measure is *opportunity cost*. This is the cost that you pay every time you make a decision. But it's not the price tag. It's the cost of foregoing your next best alternative.

For example, this morning I chose to write this chapter of this book. If I hadn't chosen to write, I would instead be training in martial arts. Therefore, the opportunity cost of writing this chapter is a few hours of training in Muay Thai. That's what I had to give up in order to write this chapter.

When I combine the truth that I'm always giving up some opportunity to do whatever I'm currently doing with the fact that I'm going to die relatively soon, it lights a fire under my belly. It gives me a clear perspective on just how valuable my time really is.

Yes, I value my friendships and my family. And yes, I value owning a nice car and other material objects. But at the end of the day, I can't allow other people or other things to trump the value of my own, ever-decreasing time.

And before you dismiss this as ego-centric, realize this means that every time I hang out with a friend, or buy a new phone or t-shirt, I'm consciously choosing to spend time doing that over doing something else.

And when you spend your money on anything, you're really spending the time that it took you to earn that money. For example, if I go to the store and buy a $1000 watch, I just spent every minute that it took me to earn that $1000 on that watch.

Again, absolutely nothing trumps the value of your own time.

Take Action

Clearly, in order to dominate life, you must value your time above all. And in order to value your time above all, you must review how you're currently spending your time.

Conduct an audit of how you spend your time over the next

week.

Each night, just before going to sleep, simply take out a note pad, or open a Word document, and jot down how you filled your time during that day. Be brutally honest. Account for every hour you were awake.

After you finish, go back through each block of time, choose the one activity you're least happy you spent time on, and write down its opportunity cost. If you didn't do that particular activity, what's the best way you could've spent that time?

This will shed light on how you can potentially make better use of your time, and assist you in better dominating life.

PART II: FEAR

There are very few monsters who warrant the fear we have of them.

- Andre Gide: French author, 1869 - 1951

CHAPTER 3

Spartacus was a Thracian by birth. The Thracians were a group of Indo-European tribes located in Central and Southeastern Europe.

While the details of his upbringing and early life are debated, it's generally agreed upon that he was a fearless mercenary who became a Roman soldier. After serving in the Roman ranks for some time, he did something that went against protocol – likely he stole something or deserted.

Thieves and deserters were turned into slaves. Due to Spartacus' remarkable strength, he was chosen to be a gladiator. He was sent to a gladiatorial school near Capua and trained to fight to the death – for the entertainment of the Roman masses.

During this time period slaves were treated poorly and lived in highly oppressive conditions. In the year 73 BC, Spartacus and about 70 other slaves plotted an escape. The plot was betrayed one evening, but rather than backing down the men seized kitchenware and any other objects they could get their hands on and used them as makeshift weapons. Their revolt succeeded, and they broke free.

They chose Spartacus to be their leader, promptly defeated a small Roman force sent after them, and then quickly moved to a more tactically defensible position on Mount Vesuvius. When Rome sent a larger band of soldiers to defeat the men and quell the revolt, Spartacus again outsmarted them. He had his men climb down the back of the mountain on hand-crafted vine ropes, before sneaking up on the unfortified camps of soldiers and killing them all.

Under Spartacus' leadership, the original band of 70 gladiators exponentially grew to a force of over 120,000 slaves. He threatened the Roman heartland of Italy before eventually being put down. These events are not remembered in history as a mere slave revolt. They're known as an all-out war: *The Third Servile War*.

Rule 3: Identify your fears

Spartacus and his initial band of gladiators were slaves meant to fight until the death for their masters.

Given this harsh reality, it's easy to wonder why they wouldn't all revolt by default. They had nothing to lose. After all, if you were meant to die as a slave, why not die trying to escape servitude?

Yet somehow the fear of punishment at the hands of their rulers outweighed the fear of death. While there had been a few prior slaves revolts in the history of the Roman Empire, none had ever grown to threaten the Italian peninsula like this one. Clearly the fear of punishment had kept the slaves in line.

But someone at that gladiatorial school in Capua, be it Spartacus or otherwise, was able to make this distinction. He was able to clearly identify his fears. He could die at the hands of another slave for the entertainment of free men, or he could die at the hands of a Roman soldier, fighting to protect other slaves and his own self-respect.

It took a gladiator, or 70, to consciously identify the exact fear that was keeping them oppressed. They were foregoing a revolt for fear of punishment, even though they were meant to die as slaves anyway. Once they had this knowledge, the decision to revolt was easy.

More importantly, once they revolted, they were able to share this realization with over 120,000 other slaves who joined them in their war against their masters.

I know that you're no slave, but you still must realize and identify any hidden fears you have that are holding you back from doing exactly what you want. It's nearly impossible to face a fear that you don't even know exists.

Otherwise, if you don't, you'll become a slave to your fears. They will effectively rule your life and set the boundaries of what you can – and can't – do. This is the mistake that the majority of so-called men make in this day in age. They never take the time to recognize what they're afraid of. Hell, they usually don't even want to admit that they're afraid of anything in the first place, because they're afraid to show weakness.

In the end, this is their Achilles heel. This ignorance to their fears is what keeps them from doing anything of note – anything that makes a difference, anything that takes balls to do.

But if you do step past this hurdle, and bring your fears to light, you can explore them on a more conscious level. Like the gladiators who recognized that they were better off dying while fighting for their freedom than dying as slaves, you too will realize that you're better off facing your fear and failing than cowering under its pressure and becoming its slave.

My Experience

After I graduated college, I began my first career job working as an implementation engineer for a software company.

A year later, I developed a clear understanding that it wasn't something I could do for a lifetime. I found little gratification in improving the efficiency of an accounting department's ability to process invoices. It simply wasn't engaging me on a high enough level.

Over the same time, I developed a love for fitness and bodybuilding. The highlight of my day was often hitting the weights after hours of staring at a computer screen in the office. The process of growing stronger and pushing my limits was exhilarating. The changes I saw in my body made this hobby equally addicting.

The idea of changing careers and becoming a personal trainer eventually found its way into my head. And I couldn't shake it. I took three months and dedicated all of my free time towards studying for the *National Academy of Sports Medicine* training certification. Then I took the test and became a certified personal trainer.

But months passed and I was still working the same software job. It wasn't until one Saturday afternoon when my buddy asked me "why haven't you changed careers yet, then?" after I explained my situation to him, that I was able to identify the fear that was holding me back.

"Because I won't make any money in the beginning, and if I fail to build a successful training business, I could go broke."

Those words replayed themselves through my head over and over again for the next few weeks. I now knew that a combined fear of failure and fear of poverty were the causes of my inaction. I identified my fears.

Within weeks I resolved to face them. I got a job at a high-class city gym where the clientele could better afford training. This decreased the likelihood of failing to build a business. I even negotiated a deal with the software company to keep me on as a part time employee, working from home. This decreased the likelihood of falling into poverty.

Because I identified my fears, I was able to move forward in a way that mitigated their chances of materializing – but only because I identified them.

Take Action

You can't dominate life if fear is holding you back from doing something you want to do. And you can't face that fear if you don't even know what it is. The first step to facing and conquering your fears is to identify them.

For every goal you've set for yourself, however big or small, ask yourself: *what's holding me back? Why haven't I accomplished it yet?*

Note: If you don't have any goals, keep reading – part 3 of this book will assist you.

For some things, fear won't play a role. For example, I haven't finished this book yet because I haven't had the time to do so.

For other things, fear will be at the center of your inaction. The Roman gladiators realized that a fear of punishment was keeping them from revolting. I realized a fear of failure was keeping me from changing careers.

Think about anything you'd like to do, that you don't currently do. Maybe it's quitting your job. Maybe it's just telling your boss to show some more respect. Maybe it's approaching more women. Maybe it's just eating better.

Whatever it is, you must ask yourself: *what's holding me back?* The answer to this question very well may be a hidden fear – one that's keeping you from doing what you want.

CHAPTER 4

In the autumn of the year 325 BC, Alexander the Great, king of the Greek kingdom of Macedon, was in the midst of his invasion of India.

At this point, the 26 year old king had already accomplished the seemingly impossible feat of conquering the entire Persian Empire, among other territories, and solidified his legacy as one of the most dominant military commanders of all time.

But India would prove to be a different beast. At first, his momentum carried on, crushing several clans in the north of the peninsula that is modern day Pakistan, crossing the Indus River, and defeating King Porus of Punjab in an epic battle where Alexander was left with several battle wounds.

But after a long string of hard fought skirmishes, the morale of his army grew weak when they approached the river Ganges. The river's width and depth would prove deadly to cross. Moreover, the army learned of a large force of men-at-arms, horsemen, and elephants waiting to attack them on the other side. His generals begged and pleaded for a return home, so the men could rest with their wives and children and recover. Alexander was hesitant, but eventually agreed.

The problem was finding an easy way back. After some deliberation, and with no obvious choice present, he decided on the Makran Desert. It would be a challenge – no army had ever succeeded in crossing it.

The result was horrific. As the journey went on, the casualties increased. Most died from the extreme heat, or the lack of food and water.

On one particular day, several soldiers gathered all of the water they could into a single helmet and brought it to Alexander to drink. He took the helmet, paused, and asked the men if there was enough for the entire army. They replied that there was not. He thought for a moment, and then proceeded to dump the water into the sand – all in dramatic fashion.

This simple, but powerful gesture is rumored to have radically improved the morale of his army. They sensed their leader's fearlessness and belief that they could make it without water. These sentiments spread. It gave them the extra edge they needed to push on for just a little bit longer.

Soon they reached an oasis and were able to replenish their supply of water. While many men died, a sizable portion of his army survived the deadly crossing.

Rule 4: Understand the causes of your fears

Alexander the Great was able to win so many victories and write his name into the history books, for one, because he had such a good understanding of the men in his military. Like any dominant leader, he could sense, and then appropriately alter, the morale and feelings of his forces.

In the above scenario, where his men were fighting against brutal heat and dehydration, he demonstrated this superior prowess. He recognized the fear of his men – an obvious one. They were afraid they were going to die before they made it home. Any of them could have told you that.

But his success was taking this one step further and understanding the cause of this fear. His men were surrounded by death. People were dying. Their livestock was dying. Their supply of water was dying. And surely there was much talk of these growing pains and causalities. Alexander realized this. He realized that the only thing on his men's minds was death. They were plagued by a sense of hopelessness. This was the cause of their fear.

He knew he must do something so powerful that it would give

his men hope. It had to fill their minds with a feeling that they could persist and make it. He had to replace the overgrown sentiments of death and hopelessness.

So when his men brought him the remaining water, to give their king a chance of surviving, he chose that moment to make his move. He took the only sign of life, and he threw it away, into the desert sands.

Yes, on the surface this may seem morbid – like it might crush any remaining hope that they had. But the fact that he was their king made it so dramatic that it inspired them. They believed that their leader was not afraid of dying. They believed he was sure that they would make it. This certainty spread through the ranks like wildfire, and the feelings of hopelessness that caused their fear of death were extinguished.

While I know that you don't have a personal army at your command, you *do* have fears that you must overcome. And the second step in overcoming your fears, after identifying them, is understanding the root of their causes.

You can't begin to make productive strides in dominating life and becoming the man you want to be until you defeat your fears. And you can't defeat your fears until you fully comprehend why you're experiencing them. Thus, you cannot ignore this powerful rule.

But most men do. Afraid to admit their fears in the first place, they shy away from any notion of their existence. And, if by chance, they are made aware of a certain fear, they do their best to ignore it. They try to deny that it's there.

You must do the opposite. You must distinguish yourself from the masses of weak men and fully embrace the reality of your fears. You must engage them on a conscious level and feel the full force of their existence. You do this by taking the time to understand their causes. Only then can you defeat them, as Alexander demonstrated.

My Experience

I'll continue my previous example about quitting my software job and changing careers to become a personal trainer. As a reminder, I was afraid I would fail as a personal trainer and potentially risk my financial security. That's what was keeping me from making the change.

But even after identifying those fears, I still hesitated. I knew *what* I was afraid of, but I didn't know *why*. And I didn't consciously find out. If I had, I would've been able to address the root cause of my fears and move forward more quickly than I did.

It wasn't until I was reading a book, *Ignite the Fire* by Jonathon Goodman, that I realized why I was afraid of failing. This was after I'd gotten my certification. The book detailed how to apply all of the knowledge of anatomy and fitness program design I'd learned over the past few months. It ran through how to conduct an initial meeting with a training client, sell them on the value of training, and keep them motivated over the long haul.

In a sense, what this book did was give me the experience of another trainer's failures and mishaps. It gave me the experience that I lacked. And that's when I realized that my fear of failure was tied to the fact that I had no real experience selling personal training and conducting training sessions.

I was afraid I would fail because I had no idea what to expect.

Take Action

Clearly understanding why you're afraid of something has its merits. It gives you the knowledge and confidence you need to face, and eventually conquer the fear. Without this understanding, you're only slightly better off than when you didn't even know what the fear was in the first place.

In order to discover the causes of your fears you must simply ask *why.*

You ask *"what's holding me back?"* when you want to find out what your fears are. The next step is to take your answer to that question, your fear, and ask *"why is this holding me back?"*

The answer is the cause of your fear. It's the real reason you're afraid of doing something you want to or embodying some quality you desire. This knowledge takes you one step closer to dominating life.

CHAPTER 5

Edward Snowden was quiet and shy growing up. His adolescent interests in areas such as Japanese anime paint a very different picture from those of the other figures of dominance we've seen thus far.

In 2004, at age 21, Snowden enlisted in the United States Army Reserves as a Special Forces recruit. He reported that he wanted to fight in Iraq because he "felt like [he] had an obligation as a human being to help free people from oppression." But a brutal fall during a training accident broke both of his legs, ending his military career before it even started.

In 2006, he began working at the Central Intelligence Agency as a systems administrator, already demonstrating his digital prowess. This gig lasted until 2009, when he left, took a Certified Ethical Hacker course in India, and began working for private contractor Dell inside a National Security Agency facility on a US military base in Japan.

Snowden's position as a systems administrator granted him access to the most secure levels of information. More importantly, he could view this information without leaving an electronic trace. Some of the things he saw left him deeply concerned.

In May 2013, he again changed jobs, this time landing at a consulting firm within a different NSA location in Hawaii. Again, he was a systems administrator, with the same untouchable level of security clearance. He later admitted that he took this job with the sole intention of gathering data on unjust NSA surveillance so that he could leak it: "My sole motive [was] to inform the public as to that which is done in their name and that which is done against them."

Before leaking any data, he shared it with fellow employees and two supervisors, even. He told them about global surveillance programs such as PRISM and MUSCULAR that monitor, collect, and store secure and encrypted data communications across the internet, effectively spying on everyone online. While the information bothered them, he says, "no one was willing to risk their jobs, families, and possibly even freedom." So he took it upon himself.

On May 20, 2013, Snowden took a leave of absence, to allegedly get treatment for his epilepsy, and flew to Hong Kong. Days later, news contacts he'd previously met with began to publish leaked documents he'd shared with them.

The US Department of Justice promptly charged him with espionage and revoked his passport. His life was immediately in grave danger. But this didn't surprise him. Snowden had already acknowledged his fate to one of the reporters with whom he shared the documents:

"I understand that I will be made to suffer for my actions."

Rule 5: Determine the worst possible outcome – and accept it

The only way you'll ever truly face any fear is to accept the possibility of the worst possible outcome. For Edward Snowden, this was death at the hands of the United States government, or one of its agents. It was the possibility that he'd have to live the rest of his life in hiding, behind bars, or six feet deep

This is an extreme example. With most fears, you'll realize that the even worst possible outcome really isn't so bad. It's rarely bad enough that you should be living in its shadow, or under its control.

The problem is that we hardly ever take the time to consciously determine what the worst possible outcome is. And we can't determine what the worst possible outcome is if we don't even know what we're afraid of. That's why this step comes after recognizing your fears, and understanding their causes.

If you've already taken the time to identify what's holding you back from dominating life and understanding why it's holding you back, then you're already leagues ahead of the average man. Your leagues ahead of the man who's so afraid of death and trying new things that he lives in his own little fantasy world where fear doesn't exist.

But before you begin the celebration – before you actually confront and conquer the fear – you must prepare yourself for the worst possible outcome. This will allow you to approach the situation from a position of strength and focus, rather than a position of weakness and fear of the unknown.

Be careful. You don't want to dwell on this outcome for so long that it fills your mind with doubt and thoughts of failure. You simply want to quickly acknowledge that it's a possibility. Then you can move on. You can focus the rest of your energy and efforts on doing your best to avoid it, and succeeding in your quest to conquer the fear.

My Experience

There's nowhere in my life that this simple concept has made a bigger impact than approaching new women. Meeting women by approaching them on the streets, at the store, or at the bar is a universal fear of man. We see a cute girl who we'd love to talk to, among other things, and then we choke up.

We fill our minds with negative thoughts about not knowing what we're going to say, or how they might be in the middle of something important that we shouldn't interrupt. We don't take the time to approach the situation with a level head.

It wasn't until I applied an approach similar to the one I preach in this book that I was able to conquer this fear and effortlessly and confidently approach attractive women:

What was I afraid of that kept me from approaching cute girls? I was afraid that they wouldn't like me, and that they'd turn me down.

Why was I afraid that they wouldn't like me? I was afraid they wouldn't like me because I thought it would be embarrassing and hurt my ego.

What's really the worst possible outcome when I approach a girl? The worst thing that can happen is that she won't like me and I won't get her phone number, or inside her pants. That's it. She isn't going to shoot me down or take my wallet. The worst thing she can do is say *no thank you*.

And then I realized that I was never better off not approaching. The worst thing that could happen is that I didn't go on a date with her. And that's exactly what was going to happen if I didn't approach her in the first place.

I'm not Edward Snowden. When I decide to approach a cute girl, FBI and CIA agents aren't going to parachute down from the skies and kill me. There's literally nothing on the line. And when I made this realization, I began to fearlessly approach women, and go on far more dates.

I conquered my fear, however irrational it was.

Take Action

In order to effectively conquer any fear, you need to acknowledge and accept the possibility of the worst outcome.

The magic of this technique is that with many fears, such as my personal example of approaching women, this step has the potential to virtually eliminate the fear entirely, before you even face it.

To put it into action you must already know what your fear is. You must know the exact thing that's keeping you from executing some action that you know you must, in order to be the man you want to be. You should also have identified and understood why this thing is paralyzing you, and stopping you from moving forward.

At this point, the next step is to ask *"what's the worst possible thing that could happen when I face this fear?"*

And once you have an answer to that question, you must accept that it very well may happen. Edward Snowden very well may suffer or die for initiating the single biggest leak of secure documents in United States history. The girl you approach very well may tell you she has a boyfriend or to get lost.

Yes, you should try to avoid this outcome at all costs, but you have to accept its possibility to confront and conquer the fear from a place of confidence and dominance.

CHAPTER 6

Robert Smalls was born into slavery in 1839 in Beaufort, South Carolina. His master decided to lease him, which led him to working a variety of jobs in the hotels and streets of Charleston before ending up at the docks.

He loved the water, and did well at the dock jobs as a result. He quickly moved through the ranks – starting as a dockworker and moving onto being a rigger, then a sail maker, and eventually a wheelman. A wheelman was another name for pilot, because blacks couldn't be called pilots.

This job led the bright Smalls to gaining a thorough understanding of the layout of the Charleston harbor. Furthermore, his skill and knowledge built a deep trust within his boss' minds. They regularly spent the night ashore, leaving Smalls and a ship full of slaves all by themselves.

One such night, in the fall of 1861, Smalls decided to take advantage of this circumstance. He created a plan to sail the boat, full of a dozen or so other slaves, including his wife, through the harbor, past Confederate fortifications, and north to the Union blockade – to freedom. If they were caught in the act, Smalls mentioned to his wife, the outcome was certain: "I shall be shot."

At 3 AM, Smalls dressed in a uniform similar to the captain's, donning his trademark straw hat to cover his dark skin. He proceeded to back the ship, the *CSS Planter,* out of the Southern Wharf. He made his way to another nearby wharf and stopped, picking up family and friends of the crew – another bold move.

With a boat full of slaves – men, women, and children – Smalls made a run for it. He used his knowledge of the harbor to avoid mines as they went. Eventually, around 4:30 AM, they neared Fort Sumter, a large Confederate fort that guarded the harbor.

Passing this was his biggest challenge. Again, he called upon his aquatic experience, this time giving a silent signal to the fort – *pass the Planter*.

They let him through. He headed straight for the Union blockade. As he approached it, he hoisted a white sheet as a flag. The first boat in the fleet, the *USS Onward,* saw the oncoming boat and prepared to fire, before seeing the white flag at the last moment.

Smalls plan succeeded. He became a free man, and brought his whole crew along with him.

Rule 6: Confront your fears

All of the previous steps we've covered – identifying a fear, understanding its cause, and determining the worst possible outcome – are important. But, at the end of the day, the only thing that's absolutely necessary is that you actually confront the fear – you do the thing that's paralyzing your action.

And that's just what our friend Robert Smalls showed us. Yes, he identified his fear, and even went to the lengths of determining the worst possible outcome – telling his wife he was aware of the deadly punishment he could face. But, more importantly, he actually faced his fear head-on and executed his plan in spite of it. If he didn't, both he and his crew would've eventually died in servitude, with nothing to distinguish themselves from the next slave.

As we saw with Spartacus and the gladiators, slavery works because of the fear of punishment. Slaves obey their masters because they're afraid that if they don't, pain or death will be inflicted upon them. And this fear is what keeps most of them in line. But some great men, like Robert Smalls and Spartacus, are able to face their fears. They're able to realize that their lives will go nowhere if they don't.

And this is no different from society today. Most men live a life confined to working at their office and watching television inside their home. They're afraid to face their fears of failure, poverty, or whatever else it might be. They often drink or do drugs to numb themselves and quell their desire to step outside of their own little box. In the end, they become a slave to their fears and live life in a state of paralysis, where they never step outside their box or try something new or different.

If you're to become the man you want to be, one who's bold, confident, and successful, you must face your fears head on. It's the only way to break free from their chains. The previous steps will better prepare you to face your fears. Carrying them out in the aforementioned order will increase the likelihood that you actually face them, as well as increasing the likelihood that you defeat them. But again, in the end, you always must face the fear in order to conquer it and continue to grow.

My Experience

My junior year of college I was considering the possibility of studying abroad in Madrid, Spain. But I wasn't sure if I wanted to.

I didn't know anyone else who was going. I'd never lived alone, or in Europe. And I was enjoying life at my Boston campus. I had friends. I participated in a lot of sporting activities. I was familiar with all the local bars and stores.

In short – I was afraid. I was afraid I would get to Madrid and be lonely. I was afraid I wouldn't meet new people. I was afraid I wouldn't make any friends. But on some level, I knew that all of this uncertainty was a sign that I should go. So I hesitated. I didn't make a decision.

Weeks passed, and the final day that they were accepting applications came. I resolved to go. I recognized the worst possible outcome – that I have a terrible 6 months and then return to Boston for my senior year, where everything will be *good* again. I could deal with that, I thought.

A few months later I was boarding my flight at JFK airport in New York. For the better or worse, I was headed to Madrid. I was to face my fear of loneliness.

Of course, this ended up being the best decision of my life. I was thrown so far outside my comfort zone that I grew exponentially over those 6 months. And I wasn't lonely for a second. I made fast friends and fell in love with the city. It was the best 6 months of my college career.

Take Action

Clearly you must face your fears in order to grow as a person and accomplish anything significant. If you never do anything you fear, you'll live so far inside your comfort zone that you'll rarely meet new people, experience new things, or achieve big goals.

Executing this is simple. Whenever you come to a difficult decision or uncomfortable situation in your life, you must take the route that makes you the most uncomfortable. This is the route that your fears are preventing you from taking.

If you take the easy path, you become a slave to your fears and cease to grow. But when you make a habit of choosing the difficult, fear-laden path, you begin to dominate life and dictate your own path. You become the ruler of your circumstances, instead of being their prisoner.

To reiterate the whole fear facing process:

First, ask *"what's keeping me from moving forward in this direction?"* and identify your fears.

Then ask *"why is this keeping me from moving forward?"* and understand their causes.

Then ask *"what is the worst possible outcome if I move forward anyway?"* and accept this possibility.

Finally, move forward in spite of the fear.

Use this simple 4-step process and begin to conquer fear after fear, and dominate life.

PART III: DIRECTION

If you do not change direction, you may end up where you are heading.

- Lao Tzu: Ancient Chinese philosopher, 6th century BC

CHAPTER 7

Growing up Jeff Bezos was, for all intents and purposes, a nerd.

If he wasn't being put to work on his grandfather's Texas ranch, he was watching Star Trek or working on his own little science experiments. One of these was a makeshift alarm he rigged to his bedroom door in order to keep his younger siblings out.

This thirst for technology and scientific information propelled him to excel in school, landing him a spot at Ivy League academic powerhouse Princeton University. He graduated in 1986 *summa cum laude,* with a Bachelors of Science in Engineering. This landed him a job on Wall Street in the computer science field.

One day in 1994, Bezos had a shocking revelation. He recently had learned about the rapid growth in internet usage. This intrigued him. More importantly, it coincided with a Supreme Court ruling that stated that online retailers didn't have to collect sales tax for purchases from states in which they lacked a physical presence. This caused a light bulb to go on inside his head.

He quit on that very day, leaving a lucrative job at a New York City hedge fund and hopping in a car to drive across the country to Seattle, Washington. He stopped at his parents' home in Fort Worth, Texas to pick up $300,000 that would fund his new idea. The rest of the way he wrote up a legendary business plan as he drove – the plan that became *Amazon.com.*

He would sell books online from his garage in Seattle. He chose Washington because of its relatively small population. This would take advantage of both the boom in internet activity and the aforementioned Supreme Court ruling.

What began as a small online bookstore grew to be the single largest e-commerce marketplace on the internet. According to

Forbes' latest billionaire rankings, Bezos is worth over $4.4 billion.

Rule 7: Create a goal

Bezos' success can be attributed directly to his ability to create a goal. He was able to start and grow *Amazon.com* into the most dominant, and perhaps profitable, website on the internet because of this crucial skill.

Today far too many people get caught up in the notion of *setting* goals. This carries a different connotation than *creating* goals. Yes, setting goals is leagues above not setting goals, but it facilitates a set of limiting beliefs.

The problem is that many people get caught up in a back-and-forth in their mind. They get frustrated because they can't think of any goals to set – and then they don't. They remain paralyzed and stagnant. They don't realize that they can simply create a goal out of thin air. It doesn't need to be somehow validated. It just needs to be.

When you think along the lines of creating a goal, it gives you the freedom to conjure up anything you want, no matter how crazy it may seem. In fact, I guarantee you that if Jess Bezos had attempted to get *Amazon.com* funded through traditional means, rather than by borrowing his parents' money (a definite advantage he possessed), he likely would have been rejected by most investors.

But this is all beside the point. You don't have to create the next *Amazon.com*. You simply need to give your life a purpose, however big or small it may be. A man without a purpose – without a direction – is impotent. He has no motivation – no driving force that he can focus his daily energy and efforts around. He can easily fall into depression.

You must avoid this trap, a trap that the majority of men fall for today. This is probably the biggest reason that so many men become complacent with their lives. They get a job and fall into a routine. They fail to re-evaluate or set a new direction for their lives. They live without purpose.

Creating a goal is the undisputed solution to this problem. It gives you direction and purpose. It doesn't matter if the goal is getting a job, getting a promotion, learning a new skill, or just facing a fear – it only matters that it exists and that you consciously acknowledge it.

My Experience

A few months ago, I realized that something was missing in my life. I created the goal of writing this book, but it wasn't enough.

Something you'll undoubtedly discover when you get in the habit of creating and achieving goals, if you haven't already, is that one often isn't enough. Your base level of motivation and drive increases to the point where you need more stimulation.

While I definitely had enough work on my plate, between writing the book, maintaining my personal training business, and putting in part time hours working as a consultant for a software company – I needed an extracurricular activity of sorts. The only thing I was doing outside of work at the time was weight lifting.

A few years ago I took Krav Maga classes, and really enjoyed them. For those of you who don't know, Krav Maga is a self-defense system created for use by the Israeli Defense Forces. It preaches only the most brutal and practical techniques.

As I thought back on my experiences there, and the various skills I learned, I realized that I was really starting to miss it. So I created the goal of learning a new martial art – one where I'd be able to spar more and learn a new set of fighting skills.

I proceeded to try out two classes at a nearby Brazilian Ju-Jitsu gym. After the two classes passed, I really wasn't hooked. But I still wanted to learn a new martial art. So I searched a bit more on Google, and decided to try a free class at a Muay Thai gym.

A few days later, I walked in. It was located in a basement. It reeked of sweat. The fighters were experienced and a bit standoffish, but the class was exhilarating. I quickly learned new techniques, got a killer workout, and got my ass beat down. But it was awesome. I signed up for a year. I fulfilled the recent goal I'd created.

Take Action

One of the most fundamental steps you must take in order to dominate life is to give yourself a purpose. You must create a goal and give yourself direction. Otherwise you'll never change. You'll never separate yourself from the depressed, content masses.

Think of it like getting into a car and driving. You have to have a destination. Otherwise you won't get anywhere – anywhere meaningful, at least.

Start by brainstorming a list of outcomes you'd like to achieve. If you're struggling, try to create a small goal for each of the following categories:

1. **Professional** (getting a job, getting a promotion, changing careers, stating a business)

2. **Physical** (losing weight, building muscle, solving a health problem, learning a martial art, participating in a sports league, complete a *Tough Mudder* type race)

3. **Adventure** (hiking a mountain, visiting an exotic destination, taking a vacation)

4. **Personal** (meeting new women, going on a date with a cute girl, finding a girlfriend, writing a book, starting a blog, taking a programming course on CodeAcademy.com, learning a foreign language)

Don't get caught up trying to create the *perfect* goal. It doesn't exist. Just choose one thing to get started with. If you have trouble, then start with something small that you can accomplish within a matter of weeks (i.e. going on a date with a cute girl, taking one martial arts class, going to the gym three times a week for a month).

Realize that it's not the specific goal that matters – it's simply the fact that you have one.

CHAPTER 8

Sean Carter was born into poverty in 1969. Growing up in the Marcy Houses housing projects in Brooklyn, he was surrounded by drugs, crime, and a culture of hopelessness. Most men ended up dead or in jail by their early twenties.

"Crack [cocaine] was everywhere," he recalls. "It was inescapable."

The early departure of his father didn't help the situation. At age 12, he shot his brother in the shoulder for stealing a piece of his jewelry. But then he got involved in a ring of up-and-coming rappers that included LL Cool J and Big Daddy Kane. Carter took on the stage name "Jazzy" and began to take part in freestyle battles, eventually becoming Big Daddy Kane's hype man and rapping in between songs at his concerts.

While he continued to create opportunities for himself, collaborating with big names such as Big L, DMX, and Ja Rule, he couldn't get any record labels to give him a shot. Carter couldn't seem to achieve the only goal he really wanted: to break into the rap game by singing a record deal.

So he took it upon himself. He began by hustling on the streets and selling crack. But he was careful not to get caught in the vicious cycle that most drug dealers fell into. "You have to have an exit strategy, because your window is very small," Carter says, looking back. "You're going to get locked up or you're going to die."

He heeded these words of caution. As soon as he had enough money, he teamed up with two friends and created his own record label: *Roc-a-Fella Records*. If no one was going to sign him, he was going to find his own way.

By creating his own label, Carter effectively cut out the middle man, and would yield more profits if he could produce an album that sold. Next he struck a deal with reputable distributor *Priority Records,* and soon released his debut album *Reasonable Doubt* under his new name: Jay-Z.

The album spread through the streets of New York City like the plague. It quickly reached number 23 on the *Billboard Top 200.* Carter had finally accomplished his goal of making a name for himself in the rap game.

Rule 8: Make a game plan

If creating a goal is choosing a destination for your trip, then making a game plan is getting the list of directions to get there. Without GPS or MapQuest, you'll likely ever arrive at your intended location. Well, you might not make it there if you rely on MapQuest, but you get the point.

While only a small percentage of men create goals for themselves these days, a far smaller percentage ever accomplish them. The ones who do usually have a game plan, they don't just create a goal and then haphazardly go for it.

Jay-Z created the goal of breaking into the rap game by signing a record deal. When his initial attempts to get signed by collaborating and making guest appearances failed, he decided to make a game plan.

Rather than continuing to bang his head against the wall and spend his time doing things that weren't working, he took a step back and thought about it. He resolved to start his own record label. And in order to do this, he would need capital. That's where the drug dealing came in. No, it's not ethical and I certainly don't advocate dealing drugs, but it was commonplace in his neighborhood and, more importantly, it worked. It was a means to an end – just a single step in his game plan.

With money in hand, he was able to create his own record label and pay *Priority* to distribute his debut album. And this process is not something Jay-z did once and forgot about. Equal parts rapper and entrepreneur, his achievements range from selling over 75 million records and competing for the title of best rapper of all time to starting his own clothing line, *Rocawear,* and creating his own professional sports management company, *Roc Nation Sports*. Clearly he understands the process of creating and achieving goals, as he demonstrated from an early age.

The main lesson to learn from Mr. Carter is that making a game plan is an essential part of achieving any goal. Without a game plan, you forfeit any control you have over achieving your intended outcome. You represent a chicken running in circles with its head cut off, instead of a calm, collected guru making strategic moves on the chess board.

My Experience

The most obvious place I must follow this procedure of making a game plan in my life is writing books. If I were to sit down and start writing, without any plan, I'm not sure what I'd end up with. I am sure, however, that nobody would buy it.

After I decide on a topic for a book, I begin my research. This includes research for the content of the book, as well as for the market segment that it will target. I continue this research until I have a clear picture of what the final product will look like.

Then I begin to form a detailed outline – the game plan. For this book, for example, the game plan involved the historical anecdotes, the rules and basic analysis around these anecdotes, the stories from my life, and the basic steps I cover in the *Take Action* sections.

The resulting game plan is easy to follow and ensures that I'll end up creating precisely the book that I want to. Without a game plan, my ideas are nearly worthless.

Take Action

As you can see, a game plan is absolutely necessary to actually achieve any goal that you create.

Don't fall into the trap of creating a goal – making a new smartphone app, for example – and then just fantasizing about how awesome it would be. I see so many of my friends and acquaintances do this all the time. They come up with a cool idea, talk about the different features it might have, and then fail to ever determine what the first step to actually making it would be.

This is why nearly every man you know never achieves anything notable. They become content with their routine life, and whenever, by chance, they happen to create a goal, it never materializes. Their inability to create a game plan leaves them in a state of constant paralysis.

To avoid this trap, you simply must make a game plan. Start by defining in detail what your goal will look like when it's fully realized. This might be the different features and screens of a smartphone app, the exact job position you desire, a specific company you wish to work for, the type of girl you want to date, or anything else.

Once you have a crystal clear image of what your completed goal will look like, you must define the steps necessary to get there. Use backward induction: start with the end goal and work your way backwards all the way until you reach a step that you can take right now.

For Jay-Z this meant acquiring cocaine. This cocaine would be sold to make money he needed to start a record label, and pay for the distribution of his first album.

For me this meant brainstorming a list of rules that I could categorize into distinct groups. Then I could begin researching impactful historical figures that embodied these rules and work towards making a complete outline.

For creating a smartphone app this might be purchasing software that can generate conceptual images of a potential app. These images could then be given to a programmer you hire to create the app.

Depending on your goal, the game plan will vary greatly. Realize that whatever your goal is, someone has likely accomplished it before. The internet contains detailed game plans for nearly any goal you can think of. If you're struggling to think of how you could create your goal, use Google. Don't fall into the trap of being average and just forgetting your goal instead.

CHAPTER 9

Floyd Joy Sinclair was born into a poor neighborhood in Grand Rapids, Michigan on February 24, 1977. Shortly after birth, his parents decided to change his name. He adopted his father's family name – Mayweather. His father's name was also Floyd, thus he became known as Floyd Mayweather Jr.

Growing up he had little choice but to pursue a career of boxing. His father was a famous boxer who fought greats such as hall of famer Sugar Ray Leonard. Two of his uncles were also professional boxers.

One day, the young Mayweather told his grandmother, who he lived with, "I think I should get a job."

She shook her head and dismissed the notion. "No, just keep boxing."

If the family influence wasn't enough to cement his destiny as a boxer, the harsh alternatives were. He'd regularly come home and see used heroin needles in the front lawn. And if that wasn't enough to scare him away from a life of crime, the facts that his father sold drugs to provide for the family and that his mother was an addict certainly were.

The young man had no choice but to pursue a life that revolved around boxing. And when his father was arrested and sent away to serve a prison sentence, boxing became an outlet for young Mayweather. Nothing helped him escape from his harsh reality like throwing jabs, hooks, and uppercuts.

Spending nearly his whole youth in the gym expecting to become a professional boxer, like those who came before him, Mayweather began to dominate from an early age. He sports an amateur record of 84 wins and just 6 losses. He even won the national *Golden Glove* championships at just 16.

His success grew exponentially as he grew, earning him a spot at the 1996 Olympics. At 19 years of age, he took home the bronze medal, but not without controversy. In his final match, he faced Serafim Todorov of Bulgaria, the eventual silver medalist. After the match, the referee raised Mayweather's hand to signal that he won. But the judges corrected him. In fact, he'd lost by a disturbingly close 10-9 decision.

The United States team filed a protest, claiming that the judges had been intimidated by the Bulgarian head of boxing officials, and that punches Mayweather had landed weren't properly scored. The decision, however, didn't change. Mayweather let everyone know what he thought in a post-match interview: "They say he's the world champion. Now you all know who the real world champion is."

This belief that he was the best propelled him forward through the rest of his career. Currently he remains undefeated as a professional boxer and is generally considered the best pound-for-pound fighter on the planet.

Rule 9: Embody the desired result

Floyd Mayweather Jr., and his rise to prominence, illustrates one important rule that you must follow in order to dominate life and consistently achieve goals: you must embody the desired result. You must behave like your goal is already accomplished, even before it actually is.

Mayweather was born into a family of professional boxers. He was surrounded by people who encouraged him and told him that he was destined succeed. All of this altered his reality. He wasn't just another kid, growing up in the projects. He wasn't just another statistic. He was a future hall of fame boxer – and he knew it.

This knowledge caused him to focus all his effort and energy into boxing. He boxed every day and was constantly improving. Nothing else was a possibility. Even when he wanted to get a part time job to make a little extra cash, his grandmother dismissed the thought and told him to keep boxing.

In the end, this laser-like focus and incredible self-belief carried him. It transformed a regular kid into possibly the greatest boxer of all time.

You must make use of the same principle. For every goal you set, you must convince yourself that it will be achieved. You must remove all doubt and any negative thoughts from your mind. You must think on only the desired result.

In self-improvement circles, they call this *The Law of Attraction*. They say that if you focus on good things happening, that the stars will align and good things will happen – that you'll attract them into your life. But it's bullshit. There's no magical law that will bring you what you want just because you think about it.

But something special does happen when you're extremely confident that you'll achieve a specific outcome. First of all, you dedicate more time and energy towards achieving that outcome, because your natural risk-averse nature is overcome – you no longer fear what might happen if you fail. Second, you begin to see opportunities you might have previously ignored.

For example, Mayweather's belief that he was going to be a professional boxer caused him to dedicate nearly all of his time to boxing. He didn't work any other jobs or spend time doing drugs. He simply boxed, and took every opportunity that came his way to compete. All of this practice led him to becoming who he is today, not some fairy godmother who granted his wishes.

Unfortunately, the average man of the day fails miserably when it comes to this rule. As we've covered, most guys don't even aspire to achieve any lofty goals at all. Of the ones who do, even fewer make a game plan to get there and ground their goal in reality. Now, we can take this a step further, because of this minority, even a smaller percentage truly believe they'll ever accomplish their goal.

No, men have become weak. But if you can muster up the confidence that it takes to believe that you'll succeed – then you likely will.

My Experience

One time when I was able to accomplish a goal by embodying the desired result came when I was looking for my first full time job. I was a senior in college, and all of my friends were also looking for work.

I've always been able to find employment in the past, so I was certain that finding my first career job would be no different. I would have a job within a few months – no questions asked.

This belief caused me to apply to hundreds of jobs online, attend numerous career fairs at my school, and go through countless interviews. After two months of this process, I was exhausted, but still hadn't received an offer. And most of my friends were in the same boat. Many of them slowly stopped applying, and eventually fell off altogether. They accepted defeat. Some planned to just get a job waiting tables or bartending after graduation. Others had no plan.

However, I was still certain that I'd find a respectable, high-paying job. So I continued to apply. I continued to interview. One day, while driving home on the highway, my phone buzzed. It was an email. It contained a job offer for a consulting position at a software company. I turned up the music and smiled – my belief was confirmed.

Within one week, I received two more offers. It was as if the flood gates had opened up. And it was all because I embodied the desired result. My confidence that the next interview would turn into a job offer led me to applying to more jobs, following up with more leads, and, in the end, getting several offers.

I achieved my goal because I embodied the desired result.

Take Action

In order to separate yourself from the masses, achieve lofty goals, and dominate life, you have to instill beliefs of success into your conscience. You must be certain that you'll succeed.

After you've created a clear image of a goal and made a game plan to get you there, it's time to ingrain this belief into your head. Realize that you've already proven to yourself that achieving your goal is possible. You did this by writing out a concrete game plan.

Now close your eyes and visualize each part of the journey, each step in the game plan – all the way until you're basking in the sunlight of the desired outcome. What do you see? What do you feel? What do you smell? Answer each of these questions and accept this as your future. It's going to happen.

At least once a day, close your eyes and remind yourself of where you're headed. This will ingrain it as a reality inside your conscience. It will begin to manifest itself in your words and in your actions. You'll become confident that success is inevitable.

Another technique that can be used in conjunction with this visualization is affirmations. Remind yourself verbally throughout the day where you're headed. Say it as if it's already done.

"I'm a world champion boxer."

"I've just been offered a well-paying job that I love."

"My book is an international bestseller."

"I'm dating a fit, cute blonde."

You get the point. Use these two powerful techniques and take on a whole new sense of self-confidence – one that will propel you to success.

CHAPTER 10

Harland Sanders was born on September 9, 1890 in a small town in Indiana. He was the oldest of three children. One evening his father came home with a slight fever. He died later that night, leaving his wife to earn the money, and Harland in charge of overseeing and cooking for his siblings. The mother soon remarried and Harland was freed to pursue of a life of his own.

By the age of 16 he'd already been in the United States Army, cleaned trains, and became a fireman. This trend continued as he left the firehouse to work on the railroad, and then returned to working at a different firehouse. He lost his job when he got into a fist fight with a work colleague. This fiasco repeated itself in his next job as a lawyer, when an argument with his client in the courtroom erupted into an all-out brawl.

Sanders streak of bad luck, and different jobs, continued as he earned further employment as a railroad laborer, life insurance salesman, founder of his very own ferry boat company, and tire salesman for Michelin Tire. He couldn't seem to find something he enjoyed doing that was also profitable.

It wasn't until 1930, when Shell Oil Company offered Sanders the chance to operate a small service station that he found his calling. But it wasn't the gasoline sales that did it for him. Calling back on his cooking experience growing up, Sanders began to cook chicken dishes for customers at the station. His fried chicken, cooked in a pressure fryer rather than the conventional frying pan, became wildly popular. It also cooked faster. He called it his *secret recipe*. It was so delicious that the state governor commissioned him as a Kentucky Colonel in 1935.

But again Sanders found his self-unemployed when World War II broke out, gasoline needed to be rationed, and the tourists he served dried up. He moved on to become a restaurant supervisor, but he couldn't shake the urge he had to sell his fried chicken. He was certain it could be a large scale success.

So Sanders began to travel the country, stopping at small restaurants left and right. He meant to sell his recipe, and take a nickel for every chicken sold. At first, few restaurants chose to adopt the Colonel's fried chicken. But as the early adopters began to see huge booms in sales, other restaurants quickly followed suit.

In 1964, Colonel Harland Sanders sold *Kentucky Fried Chicken* to a pair of Kentucky businessmen for $2 million. The corporation would grow to be an international powerhouse and one of the most successful fast food companies ever.

Rule 10: Persist until it's complete

If there's one principle that Colonel Harland Sanders embodied throughout his life, it's persistence. Losing his job never discouraged the man. He simply picked himself up by the bootstraps and tried his luck at a different occupation. He did this is again and again and again... and again.

And when he finally found something that he truly believed in – a goal he created, with a game plan to boot – he again painted us a picture of what it means to persist until something's complete.

He created the goal of a national chain of restaurants that sold his *secret recipe* fried chicken. Then he personally traveled the country and demonstrated his cooking technique to restaurant after restaurant. He didn't rest until over 600 locations had adopted the recipe, and were paying him royalties.

Had Sanders not displayed the persistence that he did, he probably would've given into poverty in his teens, after being discharged from the Army. But that wasn't his way. And if you mean to accomplish any worthwhile goal, you have to demonstrate the same persistence.

Even after you create a goal and make a game plan to get there – even after you wholeheartedly believe that you'll achieve it – obstacles are still bound to present themselves. Persistence is remaining confident and focused in spite of these obstacles. Persistence is taking a step back and adjusting your game plan to address these unforeseen circumstances.

If you simply stick to your game plan regardless of what happens as you go, you'll likely end up banging your head against a wall. If you stick to your game plan until something goes wrong, at which point you quit, you'll never accomplish anything.

Persistence is the glue that holds your plan together. When you remain vigilant despite opposition or seemingly impossible circumstances, you separate yourself from the weak men who run and hide at the first sign of a fight. You separate yourself from the losers and the quitters.

My Experience

When I graduated college, I found myself living a life void of female contact. I slowly realized I wasn't good with women. In college, I avoided this trap because of the sheer quantity of women I was constantly surrounded by. The opportunities were literally endless.

But in this new life, I'd have to step outside my comfort zone and risk rejection. Rejection is something that very few men handle well. As we covered in the chapter on determining the worst outcome possible, the prospect of rejection is enough to stop most men from ever even approaching a girl.

The few that work up the courage to actually approach a cute girl are usually met with rejection. And it's not a reflection on them. The fact is that there are so many factors in play when a man makes a move on a girl that you'll likely never know why you were rejected.

She could have a boyfriend. She could have just been fired, and be in a terrible mood. She could be intimidated. She could just be bat shit crazy – which reminds me of one particular rejection. My friend and I had just stepped into a bar, and made our way up a flight of stairs to the top level.

To get our nights started, we generally took the approach of trying to get rejected. This tended to get the fear of rejection out of our systems, so that we could proceed in a fearless manner for the rest of the night.

So I approached a group of three or four girls, tapped one on the shoulder to get their attention, and asked my favorite rejection-inducing question, "Which one of you makes the most money?"

Dumbfounded, they stared at me blankly for several seconds. Then one started towards me, with a certain look in her eye – the type of look a soldier makes when marching into battle.

"What type of question is that?!" she demanded to know.

I motioned my palm towards her, as to calm her down, and said, "I'm tired of working, so I'm out tonight looking for a sugar momma who can..."

"Get the f*** out of here!" she cut me off, walking close to me and getting in my face, like a bouncer throwing a drunk college kid out of a bar. "Seriously, that's so f****d up. You need to leave the bar."

She continued to throw a tantrum for a minute or two. I stood still, equally awed and confused, then smiled and slowly walked back to my friend. We laughed about it and had a good night.

The point is: when you're trying to meet new women, you have to persist past rejection after rejection before you succeed and find a girl you can date, or just talk to in a civil manner.

Take Action

Persistence is the final ingredient you need to ensure that you'll accomplish your goal.

However, because of the nature of persistence, I can't offer you a specific plan of action.

After you've created a goal, constructed a game plan, and visualized the result to ingrain its certainty into your conscience – expect to face obstacles. Expect to face obstacles that will cause you to question your ability to complete the plan. Don't think that you'll live happily ever after and become an instant success.

Instead of letting these roadblocks deter you from continuing, you must remain strong. Instead of letting these roadblocks drain your spirits, you must take a step back and re-evaluate your game plan.

Consider an alternate route you can take to reach your goal that accounts for this new circumstance. And then test it. You may very well have to re-evaluate a second, third, or even fourth time before you find a passable route.

PART IV: ACTION

To hell with circumstances; I create opportunities.

- Bruce Lee: Hong Kong martial artist, 1940 - 1973

CHAPTER 11

The exact facts surrounding the birth and adolescence of Miyomoto Musashi are debated. We do know, however, that he was born in the late 16th century and raised primarily by his uncles, who educated him in the ways of Buddhism, as well as teaching him how to read and write.

His father, a skilled fighter, died when he was young, but not before showing his boy a thing or two about swordsmanship. Whatever he taught Musashi left a deep imprint on the boy's character – this is certain.

One day, Arima Kihei, a traveling warrior, posted a challenge in Musashi's village. The boy was only 13 at the time, but this didn't stop him from writing his name on the challenge – he wanted to fight Kihei.

Soon a messenger came to the temple where Musashi and his family were staying, and informed him that the challenge was accepted. Shocked, Musashi's uncle hurried to meet Kihei and beg him to cancel the duel. Kihei was adamant that the only way for Musashi to be pardoned, and spare his life, was to arrive at the scheduled time and apologize.

When the time came around for the duel to take place, Musashi's uncle showed up and begged for the older fighter to spare his nephew's life. Musashi disregarded the pleas of his uncle. Without a second's hesitation, he up and charged Kihei with a 6 foot wooden staff. Kihei responded by attacking with his sword.

Musashi managed to throw Kihei to ground. He struck Kihei's head, between his eyes, and then beat him to death. Musashi emerged victorious from his first duel. He would win many more in the years to come.

Rule 11: Don't hesitate

Musashi was able to outmatch a far more experienced fighter because of his quick start – he didn't hesitate.

This would become a recurring theme in his life. He later wrote a book, *The Book of Five Rings*. While it focuses on martial arts, it's been recognized by business leaders and renowned entrepreneurs for its no-holds-barred strategies that can be applied elsewhere. It preaches always taking the advantage and using the most effective means possible:

The primary thing when you take a sword in your hands is your intention to cut the enemy, whatever the means. Whenever you parry, hit, spring, strike or touch the enemy's cutting sword, you must cut the enemy in the same movement. It is essential to attain this. If you think only of hitting, springing, striking or touching the enemy, you will not be able actually to cut him.

While this passage focuses on fighting and swordsmanship, it can be applied to any field. Its primary message is that you shouldn't be weighed down by unnecessary actions, but rather focus on only the few things that can make a big difference.

While this has implications far greater than refraining from hesitation, it definitely embodies this principle as well, for nothing will be accomplished in an efficient manner if you delay its start.

You can't wait for the perfect set of circumstances to arrive before you take action. When you apply this principle to your goals, it means that you must take the first step in your game plan right now. If you can't, then you need a better game plan – or a different goal. Don't weigh yourself worrying about things you can't alter or affect in this very moment.

When applied to other areas of your life, this principle holds the same significance. When it comes to meeting women, for example, as soon as you see one that you're attracted to, you must approach. Waiting for *the right moment* never works in your favor – it only leads to reduced confidence and second guessing.

Even with your goals, if you don't begin right now and start making progress, it's easy to question your ability to achieve the end result. Inaction never leads to anything good. The direction you've chosen for yourself is worthless if you don't act on it. You essentially have no direction. You become another one of the sheep, who only dreams of change, but never realizes it.

A final area where this rule rings true is basic decision making – something many men are afraid to do. Realize that whenever you face a tough decision, where the better choice isn't immediately clear, waiting and sitting on the fence is rarely your best course of action. It only serves to make you a less decisive person, and encourage further hesitation in your life. Moreover, people view those who struggle to make decisions as weak. When you're able to step up and make quick, hard decisions, people will instantly view you as someone powerful – a natural leader.

My Experience

As a personal trainer, I see more people's goals abandoned and left un-achieved than you can possibly imagine. And it's almost always due to inaction.

I can't count how many times I've met with a new or prospective client and helped them clearly define their goals.

"I want to lose weight," they state.

"Why?" I ask, trying to find their real motivation.

"Because I'm fat."

"And why don't you like being fat?"

"I can't fit into any of my old clothes. It makes me feel old, lazy, and worthless."

"Ahh," I say, "so if you were able to fit into your pair of jeans from your college days, how would that make you feel?"

"Strong, I guess." And they look up at the ceiling with a smile, imagining their fit, former self. "I'd feel young again. Revitalized. Potent."

And I've sold them on the value of training with me. They now have a clearly defined goal. They're no longer buying hours at the gym, but a new identity. I then present them with a game plan that will get them where they want to be. It's a simple matter of eating less, moving more, and lifting weights with me to ensure they retain their lean body mass and develop proper movement patterns. But, unfortunately, and all too often, they give up before they start.

"I need a month to take care of some work stuff."

"My wife and I need to look at the finances. I'll get back to you soon."

And maybe some of these excuses are true. But what I can tell you definitely *is* true is that I see them completely abandon their goal. They stay fat. They lose whatever motivation they had. They get fatter.

They never accomplish their goal – all because they failed to act. The game plan to lose weight was laid out in front of them – in plain sight. If they followed it, they would've accomplished their goal. But they hesitated, they lost motivation and confidence, and they failed.

Take Action

In order to avoid hesitation, you must take immediate action.

Complete the first step of your game plan and start working

towards your goal. Do it today.

Approach the next attractive girl you see. Waiting will only guarantee your failure.

Start counting your calories and start exercising. Do it every day, starting now.

Order the first item that catches your eye on the restaurant menu. This serves as practice for making tougher decisions more quickly.

When someone defers a decision to you – whether it's where to eat dinner or what time to meet – make a quick choice, *never* respond by saying that you're indifferent.

If you wait, you won't ever see results. You'll stay a slave to whatever unproductive patterns and habits you've developed over time. The only way to break free from the hordes and hordes of impotent men is to act now, and to decide immediately.

Start small if big changes are too intimidating: skip just one snack, exercise for just 20 minutes, approach just one girl, make just one phone call, write just one page, make just one small decision – just do something.

CHAPTER 12

Curtis Jackson was born and raised in the South Jamaica neighborhood of Queens, New York. He was raised by his mother, a cocaine dealer and a lesbian. She died when he was only 9, and he moved in with his grandparents.

It didn't take long for him to get involved in the street life. "When I wasn't killing time in school, I was sparring in the gym or selling crack on the strip," he recalls. At the age of 16, he was caught with a gun while walking through the metal detectors at his high school. His grandmother found out, and sent him to a correctional boot camp.

He soon left, and gave himself the nickname *50 Cent* – a metaphor for "change". At 21, he began rapping in his friend's basement, and quickly recognized his innate talent for making music. 3 years later, in 1999, a group of producers working for Columbia Records noticed him and signed him to a record deal.

But it didn't last. On May 24, 2000 Jackson was in the car with his friend. He got out to quickly fetch some jewelry from his grandmother's house. When he returned, he sat back down, and another car pulled up beside them.

A gunman got out, walked up to the left side of Jackson's car, and proceeded to empty the entire clip of a 9mm handgun through the window. Jackson was hit 9 times, including a shot to the head that split through his left cheek and left a bullet fragment in his tongue.

He was rushed to the hospital, where he made a miraculous recovery and was released just days later. The bullet fragment was left in his tongue, however, due to caution for the many nerve endings in the area. When he got out, he was informed that Columbia Records had dropped him and shelved his upcoming album. They wanted to distance themselves from the violence and controversy that now surrounded his name.

Rather than getting discouraged and giving up his hopes and dreams, Jackson proceeded to shift the bleak circumstances into his favor. He started by retreating to his girlfriend's house in Pennsylvania to recover, avoid the men that put the hit out on him, and plot his return to music.

He made a game plan. When he was fully healed, he headed to Canada, where he could record music under the radar. Jackson proceeded to record song-after-song. He reinvented himself, embracing his violent street rep and his newly realized voice, which featured a distinct hiss – a side effect of the remaining bullet fragment in his tongue.

In 2002, he independently released the product of all this plotting and hard work, a mixtape, fittingly titled: *Guess Who's Back?* The mixtape gained instant popularity and launched Curtis "50 Cent" Jackson right back into the spotlight, where'd he stay for years to come.

Rule 12: Make your own luck

Jackson was able overcome seemingly impossible circumstances and not only survive, but thrive, because of his knack for opportunism. In the bleakest of times, he sensed a rare opportunity, and then put everything he had into turning it into gold.

Most people live their lives on auto-pilot. When an unexpected opportunity comes their way – something they aren't familiar with – they ignore it or decline it. They prefer to maintain their routine ways.

50 Cent demonstrated what could be done by embracing an opportunity that most people would never even see. Yet people turn down real, obvious opportunities every day. How often do your hear a friend or a colleague tell you that they were offered that dream position in Hawaii, but chose to decline it. They just

felt more comfortable doing the same old, same old instead.

You have to avoid this trap. Whenever an opportunity presents itself, you must embrace it. It will make your life more exciting, more fulfilling, and more successful. Nobody remembers the man who took one job and stuck with it until he died, retired, or was fired. No, history remembers the bold and the brave.

You must be ready to identify a new opportunity at a moment's notice. And, more importantly, you must be prepared to embrace it. 50 Cent did this more than once. The legendary rapper has time and time again displayed this skill, producing businesses, books, movies, video games, and more. He simply doesn't let an opportunity pass him by. And that's why he's so successful.

When faced with a similar set of circumstances, the average man would've died off or faded into a dead-end life of crime and drugs. But 50 Cent didn't. We must learn an important lesson from his success. We must do the same, and take advantage of every new opportunity that presents itself.

At the end of the day, there's no such thing as luck. Luck is just a term that the weak and fearful use to describe those who take advantage of opportunities – those who aren't slaves to their routines – those who dominate life.

My Experience

While I don't have an example as striking as 50 Cent's, I certainly try to embody this principle and take on new opportunities whenever I can.

A few months ago, while I was working out, I received an email. It was an invitation to be part of a fashion show. They needed trainers to coach the models on stage as they sported the latest line of fitness apparel.

My initial instinct was to delete the email and continue my workout in peace. But I recognized this meant I'd be passing up an opportunity to do something different. So I quickly replied: "count me in."

I had no idea what to expect, but I showed up regardless. It took place at an upscale nightclub in downtown Boston. I won't go into details, but it was an experience I'm glad I didn't miss.

My time that night was split between hanging out with models, drinking free drinks, showcasing some exercises – and my muscles – on the runway, and having a crowd of college girls who attended the show competing for my attention.

Take Action

Gentlemen, you must recognize opportunities and act on them. You must make your own luck. You can't live the life of a mindless chump who passes on doing new things by default. It will be your end.

You probably don't realize how many opportunities are placed in your lap. You probably don't realize how *lucky* you could be.

To take action and begin seizing these new opportunities, you simply have to keep your eyes open. When someone asks you if you want to do something or go somewhere and your initial instinct is to pass and say no – stop. Think about it. Are you saying no because it genuinely doesn't interest you on any level? Or are you saying no because it's something new and you'd rather stay inside your own little comfort zone?

Ask yourself: what would you be doing instead? Is it something so valuable that you can't try this new thing out? Do you really have anything to lose?

Be honest with yourself. Try new things. Make your own luck.

CHAPTER 13

Jesus Navas was born in the small city of Los Palacios, located just outside of Seville in southern Spain, in 1985.

From a young age he displayed an innate talent for football (soccer), and was chosen to join the youth ranks of the professional *Sevilla Futbol Club* when he was just 15. However, his life was marked by a serious case of anxiety attacks that were triggered whenever the boy ventured too far away from home.

These attacks are overwhelming and marked by similar symptoms to those of a heart attack: a vastly increased heart rate combined with intense sensations of trepidation. They ruled his life.

Navas constantly opted to sit out of pre-season tours, where the team traveled around to other cities in the south of Spain. One time, the coaches even had to phone his father to come pick him up when he experienced one of these terrible attacks at a training camp in the neighboring city of Huelva, barely an hour away from home.

He was simply afraid. He couldn't face an outside world that he wasn't familiar with. As he aged, his skills on the field continued to improve. The national team took notice and invited him to join them abroad. Without a second's thought, Navas would turn down the offer, year after year. In 2007, his club had agreed to sell the player to the English powerhouse Chelsea, but again, Navas rejected the move – he couldn't face the unknown perils of England.

The frequent reoccurrence of the anxiety attacks coupled with the fact that they were severely limiting his potential as a football star eventually led the player to undergoing therapy. His confidence slowly increased and his symptoms slowly declined.

In 2010, he finally agreed to join the Spanish national team at the World Cup in South Africa, a long way from home. While he wasn't included in the starting lineup, he was consistently the first Spanish player off the bench, and was praised for bringing a faster pace and better passing to the team.

On July 11, 2010, during the World Cup Final in Johannesburg, Navas entered the game late. It was scoreless and tied 0-0 when he came in. With just minutes remaining in overtime, Navas got the ball in his team's own half of the field. He quickly dribbled it up field, passing defenders left and right, before beginning a string of passes that led to the winning goal.

In that minute, the once deadly homesick boy wrote his name into the history books – all because he was able to face his fear of the unknown.

Rule 13: Embrace the unknown

As we've clearly seen, hesitation is the number one cause of inaction. And inaction is the number one thing that prevents you from achieving goals, conquering fears, and becoming the man you want to be.

Possibly the largest cause of hesitation is a fear of the unknown – a sense of uncertainty. If you allow this feeling to overcome you and prevent you from taking action, you'll never be able to make the changes you desire.

Jesus Navas illustrated this principle to a *t*. He didn't know what was outside of his hometown of Seville, and he let this stop him from tackling a number of new experiences. It stunted his growth as a footballer and his development as a man.

The first time he was able to break through this uncertainty and embrace the unknown, he helped his country capture a World Cup trophy, the biggest achievement in soccer.

You too must act in spite of unknown circumstances. If you

cannot move forward without perfect information, then you'll rarely, if ever, move forward at all. Furthermore, your resistance to acting in spite of unknown variables will quickly diminish if you can just push through the urge to remain idle the first few times.

And when you couple this rule of embracing the unknown with the previous two rules of making your own luck and not hesitating, you'll begin to see rapid change and improvement in your life, your mood, your energy, and your confidence.

You'll transform into the spontaneous man who rises to every challenge and achieves goal after goal. You'll separate yourself from the herd of sheep that are afraid to stick their necks out and move in the direction of their dreams.

My Experience

Two years ago I decided I wanted to make a website. I wanted to learn how to design websites on the WordPress platform. But I couldn't decide what type of site to make.

The idea of a blog came to mind, because it would an easy first step. But then I realized this would mean sharing my writing online, where anyone could see. If I wrote about my life, my opinions, or my experiences, they would be put on display for friends, family, co-workers, and strangers to read.

This notion filled my mind with uncertainty. Who would see it? How would they react? Would there be negative consequences?

After a bit of deliberation, my desire to experiment with web design got the best of me and I purchased the **www.HowToBeast.com** domain name.

For the first few weeks, I wrote nothing. I just focused on the design aspects of the site. Then I started to write. And I loved it. I'd never written outside of academics, but it was exhilarating. Thoughts quickly came to my mind, and I learned things I didn't know about myself as I went.

But I didn't share it with anyone except my brother. I didn't know how they'd react. I couldn't embrace the unknown... until I did.

Little by little, I shared the blog with my friends and family, who in turn shared it with other friends and family. And something powerful happened. Yes, I got comments, compliments, and questions about it, but something more powerful than that occurred.

I developed an incredible resistance in my character. All of a sudden, I honestly didn't care what other people thought about me. I didn't care who knew about the site. My confidence shot through the roof along with my ability to embrace the unknown.

Take Action

Your ability to act in the face uncertainty and embrace the unknown will have a large impact on your ability to take action and move forward as a man.

You must not let a lack of perfect knowledge deter you from trying something new, or changing something about yourself. If you do become a slave to this uncertainty, you'll never dominate life and become the confident man you want to be.

You must realize when you find yourself stalling because of a fear of the unknown. You must recognize that this is the cause of your hesitation. And because we're dealing with a fear of sorts, you must follow the steps laid out in Part II of this book:

What's stopping you from moving forward? In this case, it's the presence of a large degree of uncertainty.

Why is this uncertainty stopping you from moving forward?

What's the worst possible outcome that could occur if you move forward anyway?

Finally, accept this possibility, embrace the unknown, and go crush whatever obstacles lay in your path.

PART V: OWNERSHIP

Most people do not really want freedom, because freedom involves responsibility, and most people are frightened of responsibility.

- Sigmund Freud: Austrian neurologist, 1856 - 1939

CHAPTER 14

John Fitzgerald Kennedy won the 1960 presidential election. After serving in the military, as a Senator, and as a Congressman for the previous 13 years, he finally reached the pinnacle of United States politics and became president. As most presidents do, he inherited a number of disturbing problems.

One of these problems was Cuban Prime Minister Fidel Castro and his rise to power over former US-friendly leader President Fulgencio. Castro had already broken economic ties with the US and begun building a relationship with the Soviet Union. This scared US officials, as the country was in the midst of the Cold War with the Soviets, where nuclear tensions were quickly rising.

United States President Dwight Eisenhower, who preceded Kennedy, had begun to take action against Cuba, appropriating over $13 million to a covert CIA operation that would overthrow Castro. The plan was to train and arm a large group of Cuban exiles, who would then invade Cuba and eliminate Castro.

When Kennedy recited his oaths and took office, the plan was already in motion. A force of over 1400 exiles had been recruited, trained, armed, and was awaiting orders to attack from their current position in Guatemala. Kennedy approved the plan and authorized the offensive.

On April 13, 1961, the troops shipped out. They were split into five infantry battalions and one paratrooper battalion. Two days later, before they arrived, a force of eight B-26 bomber jets, supplied by the CIA, attacked nearby Cuban airfields. Two days later, the troops landed on a Cuban beach, Playa Giron, in the Bay of Pigs.

After three days of deadly combat, they were forced to surrender. The offensive failed miserably.

Kennedy's administration was embarrassed, having failed so badly, so early in their tenure at the White House. To add to the distress, reports began to surface that Soviet KGB officials discovered the plan and communicated it to Castro before the attack was even launched. If this wasn't bad enough, the CIA was suspected to have known about these reports, yet failed to inform the President.

But Kennedy didn't resort to finger-pointing. Instead, he stood up and took all of the blame for a fiasco that was ultimately his responsibility: "There's an old saying that victory has a hundred fathers and defeat is an orphan ... Further statements, detailed discussions, are not to conceal responsibility because I'm the responsible officer of the Government."

Shockingly this statement wasn't met with hate or negative sentiments, but rather widespread praise and a jump in his approval rating to an impressive 83 percent.

Rule 14: Own your successes and your failures

One of the biggest mistakes a man can make is not taking responsibility for his actions. This could mean attributing his success to – or blaming his failure on – another man.

When you do either of these things, you strip yourself of the power to create your own circumstances. This is toxic. It encourages you to avoid growing, changing, or doing things that you want to, because the results aren't under your control. It reinforces the incorrect belief that altering your life is out of your hands. You avoid viewing yourself as the leader and director of your own life. You become a helpless effect of your life instead of the driving force behind it.

You effectively castrate yourself, and hand your balls over to someone else.

On the other hand, when you step up and take the blame for something that went wrong, in which you were involved, you take control of the situation. You view it through a lens that allows you to analyze what went wrong and determine what you can do differently the next time a similar situation arrives. By bringing an event or circumstance into the locus of your control, you're able to actively manage it and learn from it.

This is a powerful technique. When you begin to execute it on a regular basis, you start to feel in control of your life and make more, and better, decisions as a result.

John F. Kennedy demonstrated a second vital benefit of taking responsibility – the effect it has on other people's perception of you. Instead of doing what the average man would've done and blaming the failure of the Bay of Pigs on the CIA and misinformation, Kennedy stepped up and took the blame. He said "my bad" and people loved him for it. They respected him. They felt safe under the direction of a man who wasn't afraid to make tough decisions and admit to failure.

This same principle applies to all of us. When you see someone take the blame for something that went wrong, you also unconsciously associate that person with power. You connect their admission of blame with the concept that they were in charge of the situation in the first place.

When you take responsibility in your life, the same phenomena will occur. In addition to the positive internal benefits, people will respect you for it. And it also will create an environment where people will recognize your successes, having already come to the conclusion that you're a man of power, with the ability to make difficult decisions.

My Experience

As April rolls around again, tax season is in full swing.

Last year was the first that I published and sold my books for a profit, so I was unsure how I'd report the proceeds to the IRS and pay taxes on them.

After a few hours of Googling and messing around with *TurboTax*, I faced a harsh reality – selling books through *Amazon.com* qualified me as self-employed. Even though they made the deposit into my bank account, I effectively created the product, set its price, and marketed it. I was effectively operating as a business of my own.

That doesn't sound so bad, but it led me to having to pay a host of other taxes, fill out numerous other forms, and pay the government a hefty sum of money that had already found its way into my personal bank account.

My first instinct was to yell "Why me!? F*** the IRS, they're just criminals and thieves. Blah blah blah."

But I stopped myself and thought for a minute. I realized that this situation was caused by my decision to begin writing and selling books, something that's been immensely profitable for me. The IRS and their rules exist, for the better or for the worse. It's up to me to learn them or pay an accountant to deal with it, and then pay what I owe. This was simply a necessary step in continuing down a path that I deliberately chose.

After some research, I quickly found ways to write off expenses and save myself a lot of money. I also came to the conclusion that if I keep better financial records for purchases and costs relating to my *business,* I'll be far better off next year, when I'll have a lot more income to report.

Take Action

The benefits of admitting your failures and owning them, the same way you own your successes, far outweigh any costs it may incur. You'll quickly gain influence and power in your own life, as well as the lives of the people around you. This is a crucial step in dominating your life and emerging from the masses of weak, fearful men.

To put this rule into practice, you simply have to catch yourself passing blame. Anytime you find yourself saying or thinking any of the following items...

I can't believe this happened to me.

Why did this happen to me?

How could this happen to me?

Who screwed up?

This is unfair.

Why me?

...you must stop yourself. Continuing down any of these paths will only lead you to playing the weak role of the victim and avoiding taking responsibility. You must replace these thoughts with the following questions...

What did I do that caused this?

What could I have done to avoid this?

How did I play a part in this outcome?

What can I do next time a similar situation arrives?

Answer these questions. Accept your part in the problem. If anyone else is involved, tell them that you're at fault.

Do these things and watch as the power grows inside of you. Watch as people respect you more and more. Watch yourself become dominant.

CHAPTER 15

Jackie Robinson was born in 1919 to a large African American family living in Georgia. They moved to Pasadena, California when he was just 1. Growing up Robinson dominated a number of sports, despite being excluded from many opportunities because he was black. This success led him to attending UCLA and achieving numerous athletics feats across baseball, track and field, basketball, and football.

He even began a career for a semi-professional football team in Honolulu after graduating, but in 1941 the Japanese attacked Pearl Harbor, and the United States was pulled into World War II. Robinson was drafted and assigned to a segregated, all black unit. After refusing to sit in the back of the bus, he underwent a series of court-martial proceedings that kept him from deploying overseas and seeing any combat.

When the war ended, he chose to continue his athletic career, this time playing professional baseball for the Kansas City Monarchs, a team in the segregated Negro League. But he wanted more, so he attended a Major League tryout for black players at Fenway Park in Boston. Although the attendees were limited to management officials, Robinson was met with an onslaught of racial epithets and insults. He left embarrassed and humiliated.

But opportunity again knocked at his door when club president Branch Rickey of the Brooklyn Dodgers was looking for possible players from the Negro Leagues to augment his squad. In an interview with Robinson, Rickey asked Robinson if he could deal with the racial degradation that would come as part of the potential move and not respond violently.

Distraught, Robinson asked, "Are you looking for a Negro who is afraid to fight back?"

Rickey denied the notion and replied that he needed a Negro player "with guts enough not to fight back."

Robinson agreed, abandoned the Negro Leagues, and played a year for their Minor League team before being called up to play in Brooklyn in 1947, becoming the first black since 1880 to play baseball in the Major Leagues. He was met with intense racism and criticism.

The St. Louis Cardinals threatened to strike if Robinson was allowed to play. Furthermore, he was regularly the victim of dirty play – one time, earning him a seven inch gash in his leg. Another time, the Philadelphia team manager yelled out at Robinson from the dugout. He called him a "nigger" and encouraged him to "go back to the cotton fields".

But Robinson was strong in the face of this overwhelming opposition. He competed in 6 World Series, 6 All Star games, and was awarded both the Rookie of the Year and the National League Most Valuable Player awards. After he retired, he was inducted into the Baseball Hall of Fame, cementing his legacy as a legend.

Rule 15: Don't allow the opinions of others dictate your own self-worth

If Jackie Robinson was merely an average man, the racial degradation he faced would have gotten the best of him when he was just a kid. During the racially charged era he grew up in, many whites wanted blacks to believe they were worthless. They wanted them to believe that they belonged in the cotton fields, working as slaves.

Many blacks gave in to these sentiments, joining gangs and resorting to violence to prove their worth. They allowed other people to dictate what they were worth, rather than creating and owning their own value. Even a young Robinson reportedly joined a gang after being excluded from youth sports. Luckily, he was dissuaded by a friend who recognized his true potential.

While humans have grown to be more *civil*, and outright acts of racism and bullying are illegal, we still face a rough world. Many people will attempt to tell you what you can – and can't – do. It might happen subtlety, when your boss rejects your request for a promotion. Or it might be in your face, when a "friend" or acquaintance insults you or tells you that you can't do something.

Jackie Robinson faced this opposition on a grand scale. He listened as fans, owners, players, and, at times, seemingly the whole world, told him that he couldn't play professional baseball. They told him he was nothing – to give up and go home. But he owned his own self-worth. He believed that he was more than just another black man. He believed that he could compete, and dominate, the highest levels of sports. And he did.

You must do the same. You must decide what you're worth. You must decide how the world will perceive you. If you allow other men's judgments to degrade you and crush your confidence, you're no better than the next man – because most men do fall to the ground at the hands of their peers. Or their bosses. Or their co-workers. Or some strangers on the streets.

Somebody tells them that they're a worthless piece of trash, on some level, and they believe it. They accept their inadequacy and fall to their knees. They allow someone else to determine their confidence level. You must resist these attempts and realize that you alone have power over what goes on inside your head. You alone determine what you're worth. You alone are responsible for your levels of confidence.

My Experience

I was entering into my senior year of university. I studied abroad in Madrid the previous year. During that time I worked an internship where I befriended a bodybuilder. His love for weightlifting was contagious. By the time I returned to the states,

I was hooked.

While I previously lifted weights on and off, I never followed any type of plan. I came back determined. I followed an organized gym routine, tracked my strength gains, and counted my calories so I could gain weight and add mass to my skinny frame.

And it was beginning to work. I was starting to see results. But I wasn't the Hulk yet. And so when I returned to school, with my jars of protein powder, amino acids, and pre-workout supplements, I was met with ridicule from my roommates.

"You're not even big," they said, laughing and poking fun at me. No, they weren't overtly trying to diminish my sense of self-worth, but this is the kind of subconscious message that many men take to heart. They sense someone else's disapproval, and they alter their course. They allow their self-worth to be degraded. They lose confidence.

But, on this occasion, I was stalwart. I shrugged off their comments and I stuck to my guns. As time went on, I built more and more muscle. I succeeded in my quest, despite the pressure to discourage myself and allow another man's opinion to get the best of me.

Take Action

Clearly any dominant man must remain vigilant in the face of adversity in order to prevent his self-confidence and self-worth from being torn down by other men.

However, you must be careful. You cannot indiscriminately ignore other men every time they tell you something you don't want to hear. Many times our friends and colleagues have valuable advice and feedback that will help us grow and prosper.

What you must do is separate the feedback from the hate. When someone tells you something that initially comes off as negative – stop and think.

Is this good advice meant to assist me? Is it simply disguised as tough love?

Or is it a malicious attempt to subvert my efforts and intentions? Is it stemming from a sense of hate, jealously, or envy?

Once you ask yourself, and answer, these questions, it will be clear whether their words should be heeded or ignored. If it's good advice, just expressed in a harsh tone, thank them and think of how you can apply it. If not, renounce them for their attempted sabotage, or, better yet, simply turn your cheek and ignore the haters.

Realize that they very well may not consciously be trying to degrade your sense of self-worth, as they were with Jackie Robinson. They may simply be reacting to a difference in your character that makes them uneasy or afraid of what you may become.

Recognize these key indicators, respond appropriately, and continue to dictate your own self-worth.

CHAPTER 16

Kanye West was born on June 8, 1977 in Atlanta, Georgia. When he was just 3, his parents divorced. His mother assumed custody and they moved to Chicago, Illinois. Growing up, Kanye went against the grain of the common inner city black youth in Chicago, choosing to pursue his interests in art and poetry rather than sports or crime.

He excelled in school and was accepted to Chicago's American Academy of Art, before quickly transferring to Chicago State University. Before his freshman year was up, he again went against the grain, dropped out, and decided that he'd rather pursue other opportunities.

His mother recalls this incident, and what it said about Kanye: "It was drummed into my head that college is the ticket to a good life... but some career goals don't require college. For Kanye to make an album called *College Dropout* it was more about having the guts to embrace who you are, rather than following the path society has carved out for you."

Kanye decided he wanted to break into the rap industry as a producer and began creating beats for Chicago area rappers over the next few years. His break came in 2000, when he began to work with Roc-A-Fella records. His production was featured on Jay-Z's critically acclaimed album *The Blueprint*, and people often credit Kanye with revitalizing Jay-Z's career as a result.

Having conquered his goal of becoming a successful producer, Kanye adjusted his sights – he was now determined to make a name for himself as a rapper. But record companies had already labeled him as a producer. One by one, all the major labels shot him down, encouraging him to keep doing what he was good at and making beats. Furthermore, his relatively clean image didn't vibe with the popular gangsta style of the time.

But again Kanye made it his mission to redefine himself. After falling asleep behind the wheel and nearly dying in a car accident in late 2002, and in similar fashion to 50 Cent, West created his own opportunity by recording a song that would take the rap world by storm. Rapping with his jaw still wired shut, a result of the surgery that saved his life, Kanye released a mixtape featuring *Through the Wire,* a song that detailed his car crash and the aftermath. The mixtape blew up and Roc-A-Fella signed him to a record deal in 2002.

He was an instant success. His premier album, *College Dropout,* had a strong theme: "Make your own decisions. Don't let society tell you, 'This is what you have to do.'"

This was a message that West continued to embody as he continued to grow. Each of his subsequent albums was a departure from the previous. They all embodied a distinct new style. And each one set the bar higher and higher for other rappers, who always seemed to begin to emulate Kanye's most recent sound, just before he switched it up and created a new trend.

Not one to give in to success, Kanye again adjusted his sights, this time aiming at the fashion world. His initial line of clothes was canceled before its release. His next line premiered at the 2011 Paris Fashion Week. It was met with negative reviews and intense criticism. Fashion designers urged the hip hop star to stick to his strengths and forget clothing. But, somewhat expectedly, this only made West want it more.

The following year he came back to Paris with a new line, and this time it was well received. Critics applauded his improvement, and once again Kanye defied being defined by one aspect of his life.

Rule 16: Create your own identity

Kanye West has a large number of vocal critics to this day. His in-your-face, I-do-what-I-want attitude simply facilitates a strong hate-him-or-love-him relationship with the public.

I love him. All of his work aside, he's perfectly illustrated time and time again that he owns his life. He won't let his friends, fans, corporations, or anybody else dictate what direction he'll take next. He simply chooses his own path – and sticks to it, regardless of the opposition.

And that's one reason why so many people can't stand him. They watch him evolve and do whatever he wants to, and their own insecurities are immediately brought to the surface. They realize they're living a life that society chose for them. They're just doing what's expected. And they don't want to be reminded of it.

You must do as Kanye did. You must create your own path. If you let other people tell you how to live your life, then, in the end, is it even really yours?

People will encourage you to do the same as they did. They'll tell you to go to college, get a 9-5 job, get married, have kids, and buy a house. But is that what you really want? If it is, that's fine. At least be sure to choose a career you enjoy and a woman that will support you. But for many people, this "American Dream" lifestyle simply isn't what they truly want.

Today's world holds endless opportunities and endless possibilities. As you live your life you should keep your eyes open and allow yourself to deviate from the standard path when you see something you want to go after – a different path you want to follow.

If you let the opinions of others dictate what you do, you'll live in an eternal state of resentment, always wondering what could've been. You'll fade into the background and become just another statistic – another person who simply was, but never did. You'll never dominate life. You'll never become the man you truly want to be.

My Experience

After graduating from college, I began working at a software company. It was a "good" job that paid well.

And at first, I loved it. I was learning a plethora of new skills, and was being challenged every day. But it began to grow stale. I began to realize that being confined to sitting behind a desk for the majority of my life wasn't something I wanted.

I shared these feelings with my parents and friends, who mostly encouraged me to "stick it out" for another year or two and then look for a different company, where things would be different. But they failed to understand what I was looking for. A simple company change wouldn't do it. I wanted a different lifestyle. So I began to explore my options.

After months of deliberation, I decided that personal training was my next venture, something that seemed like an awful choice to everyone else. It wasn't a traditionally accepted "good" career. "You don't even need a diploma to work at some gyms," they told me.

But I couldn't shake the urge. I reasoned that if I failed to make a living training, I could always return to a well-paid software job. So I studied, got my training certification, acquired a job at a high class gym, and quit my software job – at which point they offered me a position working part-time from home. Seeing this as an opportunity to remain financially stable, I accepted.

I began working part time as a trainer and part time as an implementation engineer. I created my own path.

Take action

In order to dominate life and do what you want, you have to avoid the trap of allowing others to set the boundaries of what you can – and can't – do. You have to realize that you're the only one in control of your future, and that the categories that other people place you in aren't permanent.

They might urge you to stay in a certain category because they're jealous, and afraid to see you rise up and change. Or they might do this because they're simply more comfortable relating to you in a certain capacity. If you change, they're concerned they might lose the connection they share with you.

Either way, you can't let them hold you back. To ensure that you put this principle into action, the next time you consider doing something different, like changing careers, moving, or trying a new hobby, ask yourself the following questions:

Is this something I truly want to do?

Why do I want to take this course of action?

If I didn't have to explain myself to anybody (and you shouldn't), what would I do?

What's holding me back from making this decision?

Once you've considered and answered each of these questions, it should be clear to you what it is that you want to do – what path you want to take, what identity you want to assume.

PART VI: PRESENCE

We convince by our presence.

- Walt Whitman: American humanist, 1819 - 1892

CHAPTER 17

Cassius Clay was born in Louisville, Kentucky in 1942. One day, when he was just 12, he had his bike stolen from him. When a policeman, who also happened to be a boxing coach, encountered the boy, young Clay told the officer he was going to find the thief and "whup" him. The officer told him he better learn how to fight first. Clay took this advice to heart, and grew to be the greatest boxer of all time. He changed his name to Muhammad Ali in the process, to better reflect his adoption of the Islamic faith.

Ali possessed an incredible set of skills in the ring, such as his pristine footwork. He would flutter back and forth, lulling his opponent's conscious mind into a sleep-like state where they'd initiate poorly timed attacks that he could counter mercilessly. His style was distinct. But it wasn't his tangible skills that set him apart – it was his unmatched presence.

Early in his career, he'd regularly predict in what round he'd knockout his opponents, and then announce it publically. If this wasn't enough, he began to belittle his opponents and pick them apart. For example, he called Doug Jones an "ugly little man", and Henry Cooper a "bum" before their respective fights. He even declared that Madison Square Garden was "too small for me".

This audaciousness made him highly controversial. Most writers and boxers developed a strong disdain for Ali. But it worked. His words struck a chord with each of his opponents, who grew to fear him before even meeting him in the ring, where he cut them down and defeated them, one-by-one.

As he won more and more bouts, Sonny "The Big Bear" Liston, the reigning heavyweight champion, took notice. A date was set for their match. Liston was an intimidating figure himself, with a criminal past and strong mob ties. But this didn't faze Ali. He continued his regular act, and attempted to strike fear into the heart of Liston. He contorted his nickname and called him "the big ugly bear", noting that "Liston even smells like a bear", and promising that "after I beat him, I'm going to donate him to the zoo".

The night of the fight, Liston was furious and ready to win the match and defend his title, as he was expected to. When the bell rang for the first round to begin, he charged Ali, clearly showing his emotional response to the taunts and insults. Ali, on the other hand, was calm and confident. He skillfully dodged "The Big Bear's" initial string of exaggerated swings, before delivering a flurry of successful punches to end the round. Ali was in his head.

After six rounds, Ali was declared the winner, when Liston quit due to an injured shoulder. Ecstatic, Ali ran to the edge of the ring, pointed at the press, and yelled "eat your words!" He'd earned the heavyweight title. And, in victory, his presence remained undeniable.

Rule 17: Establish a psychological foundation of success

Muhammad Ali demonstrated the power of maintaining a psychological presence. He believed he was the best, he believed he was going to win every fight, and, in the end, this worked wildly in his favor.

His aggressive trash talk instilled a burning image of a fearless warrior into both the minds of his opponents and his own mind. His opponents saw a man that was certain he would win, and this scared them – it threw them off their game and gave him an edge. At the same time, and equally importantly, this trash talk convinced Ali himself that he was the superior boxer. He talked himself into believing he would win, and this translated into enhanced confidence and performance in the ring.

Trash-talking your way through life is hardly a good idea. Just imagine how many job offers you'd get if every time you went in for an interview you commented on how you were "too good" for "such a measly company". It would be a hilarious sight to see, but it simply wouldn't work.

Nevertheless, there's an important lesson we can all learn from Ali – establishing a strong psychological presence is incredibly beneficial to any man who wants to dominate his own life. Creating, and maintaining, a psychological presence serves to reinforce your self-confidence and belief that you can achieve or do something that's perceived as challenging, or impossible, even.

If you approach a difficult situation with an uncertain mind, then your chances of success will be greatly diminished. This mental uncertainty will bleed though in your actions and hurt your overall performance.

If you approach a difficult situation with a confident mind, however, your chances of success will be greatly improved. This mental certainty will be ever present and it will enhance your overall performance.

Ali demonstrated this in his match against Liston. He was considered an underdog, with only a tiny chance of winning. If he accepted the public expectation, and entered the ring thinking he was destined to lose, he would have lost. But he didn't. He didn't allow the expectations of other people to set his own expectation. No, he did the opposite and talked himself up. He declared that he would donate his opponent's body to the zoo after he won. He convinced himself that success was inevitable. And it came true.

You must do the same. You must convince yourself that the odds are always in your favor, even when they're not. Too many men are pessimistic and allow thoughts of defeat and worthlessness to cloud their minds. They allow these negative thoughts to take over, and in the end, they suffer because of it. They can't confidently approach women, because they're sure that rejection is imminent. They struggle to get a job, because they're intimidated by the interviewer. They don't start a training regimen or diet, because they know that they won't stick with it.

You must take the opposite approach. You must believe that the girl you're about to approach is dying to talk to you, that the interviewer will be impressed by your performance, and that your new workout plan will transform you into a shredded beast. Only then will the odds be in your favor. Only then will these outcomes come true.

My Experience

Growing up, basketball was always my sport. And my basketball career had definite ups and downs. Sometimes I believed I was god's gift to earth, and those were the times I would dominate the court. Other times I was afraid to even touch the ball, in fear that I would just turn it over to the other team.

It wasn't until I understood the principle that Ali illustrated that I was able to harness it and use it to my advantage. Unfortunately, this came after my hopes of playing ball in college failed to materialize.

It happened during a competitive men's summer league a couple years ago. I'd recently read a book that preached the importance of positive affirmations. So, before each game, I'd remind myself that "I'm the best player on the court" and that "I can score at will". If I ever began to struggle during a game, I'd tell myself these things again and again.

And it worked. My confidence was through the roof, game after game. I was able to control and maintain it, because whenever it began to waver, I reminded myself just how good I was. The car ride to the gym was my own little version of Ali's press conferences where he issued taunts and warnings of his imminent victory.

My belief that I would succeed at each game materialized in the form of increased confidence and enhanced performance on the court. I built a psychological foundation that all but guaranteed my success.

Take Action

We must all do as Ali did. We must all convince ourselves that we'll win, whether it means in the ring, on the court, in the office, or at the bar. We must believe that success is inevitable.

You simply need to remind yourself, verbally and mentally, of your competence. Whatever your situation is, create a phrase that you can use to do this.

If you're about to enter an interview, it might be: *I'm more-than-qualified for this position. I'm going to 'wow' this interviewer and get the job.*

If you're about to approach a cute girl, it might be: *Women love me. I'm attractive and confident. This is going to be too easy.*

If you're about to confront someone about an emotionally charged situation, it might be: *I will remain calm in the face of any threats or insults, diffuse the tension, and get to the bottom of this situation.*

The possibilities are endless. Telling yourself something like this over and over will embed it as a reality in your subconscious mind – you'll truly believe it – and this is why it works.

Take advantage of this simple technique, create your own affirmations, repeat them often, build a strong psychological foundation, and begin to approach life with a new sense of confidence.

CHAPTER 18

Vladimir Lenin is one of the most controversial historical figures of all time. He was born in 1870 to a wealthy family living in a small Russian city. When he was 17, his brother was executed for his involvement in the attempted assassination of the emperor of Russia, Tsar Alexander III. This planted a seed in his mind that would grow and evolve, transforming Lenin into an extremist revolutionary who would forever change the face of Russia and alter the history of the world.

Lenin began by earning a law degree and educating himself in the ways of radical politics, which eventually landed him a 3 year punishment by exile to Siberia. A few years later, in 1902, at the *Second Congress of the Russian Social Democratic Labor Party*, Lenin would begin to establish himself as a dominant leader.

The revolutionary socialist party was at a crossroads. Julius Martov, one senior party official, stated that he believed all party members should be able to express their beliefs independently of the party leaders. Lenin vehemently disagreed, arguing that the party needed strong leaders with absolute control. Realizing he had a slight majority, Lenin took this opportunity to cement his position as the head of the party. He announced that his supports were now the *Bolsheviks*, or majoritarians, and placed himself at their helm.

A few years later, while Lenin was living in Western Europe, intense social unrest across the Russian Empire led to the *Revolution of 1905*. The revolution failed, but it gave Lenin and the Russian socialist revolutionaries more ammunition to support their cause.

After the *First World War*, in February 1917, Russia again rose up in revolution, this time succeeding and overthrowing the Tsarist monarchy. On April 16, 1917, Lenin returned to Russia.

He arrived, just before midnight, at Finland Station in Petrograd, and was met by a large crowd of workers and soldiers, hosting red flags to celebrate the occasion. They were exhilarated to see one of their most renowned political exiles return home.

But Lenin was not as pleased as they were. He stepped off the train and began to deliver a shocking, yet still charismatic speech on the international impact of Russia's revolution, repeatedly stating that their work was just beginning. The crowd was expecting a simple celebratory speech, but that was not Lenin's style.

Lenin continued to practice what he so confidently and overtly preached. Just months later, he played a leading role in orchestrating the *October Revolution*, a series of events that led to the overthrow of the provisional government and the establishment of the *Russian Socialist Federative Soviet Republic.* It was the world's first socialist state – and Lenin assumed absolute control.

Over the next 7 years, he maintained this control. He made widespread reforms that were extremely popular. He also made a point to rule with an iron fist, ordering a series of mass executions that became known as the *Red Terror.* Among its victims were the previous royal family and a number of former government officials. In 1924, Lenin died after suffering a third stroke.

Rule 18: Build a strong physical presence

At first glance, it might seem strange that Lenin is my example for building a physical presence. That is, of course, until you realize that he was able to single-handedly sway politics and generate unmatched social momentum throughout the massive Russian Empire for years on end, all while standing at a measly 5 feet 5 inches tall. And he often expressed his dominance in the form of charismatic speeches that brought thousands of people to their feet – a rare feat for someone of such a small stature.

Look at any photos or video footage of this near-midget and you'll likely fail to sense his lacking height. You'll instead notice his deadly stare, strong posture, and authoritative body language. His height, or lack thereof, is probably the last thing you'll notice.

His image is so powerful that it was used to rile up the Russian people and evoke strong feelings of nationalism on posters and propaganda for years after his death. When he died, his body was even put on display in the heart of Russia at Red Square, where nearly a million people came to see it and pay their respects, in only a matter of days. Its impact was so powerful that they chose to embalm it. Till this very day you can go to Red Square and view Lenin's striking corpse. His physical presence remains strong, even in death.

You must take advantage of the same principle that allowed Lenin the power to move an entire nation. You must build a strong physical presence. And a strong physical presence is rooted in good body language.

Unfortunately, the majority of men today slouch or slump forward, and more closely resemble the figure of a nervous hump-back than a proud, confident man. And they carry this same weak mentality.

Studies have shown that adopting strong, tall body language and taking up a lot of space directly leads to more mental confidence. This means that when you assume the posture of a strong man, not only will other people perceive you as such, but you'll also assume a matching mindset. You take on the character that your body portrays. Our thoughts and our bodies simply cannot be separated – we're built to operate as a single unit.

My Experience

Again I'll call upon my experience as a personal trainer, where I've had the opportunity to assist many people in improving their posture. They always come to me with the goal of losing weight or building muscle, but when, after a month or two, I ask them what changes they're noticing, it almost always comes back to body language.

"My wife swears that I've grown two inches."

"All of my colleagues at work say that I look much more confident throughout the day."

"I've only lost a couple pounds, but everyone says I look way better. Why do you think that is?"

It's because you're finally standing up straight.

One key part of my program design, which I usually don't delve into detail about with new clients, is corrective exercise. This means assessing which of their muscles are relatively weak, and which are relatively tight.

The most common example of this is the rounding of the upper back. People work at desks, typing away with their arms in front of them all day, and this creates tight muscles across the front of their body – the chest, the front of the shoulders, and the biceps – for example. This is the cause of the common slouching posture that you see on nearly everyone today.

What I do is help them stretch out the chest and open up their posture, while focusing on strengthening their back so that they can maintain this correct posture. This is why after just a few weeks, people that came to me looking afraid and weak now appear strong and confident. No, they haven't lost a significant amount of weight or put on more than a couple pounds of muscle, they simply improved their posture. They usually reflect this change in their demeanor and their mentality, too.

Take Action

Clearly building a strong physical presence has its benefits. You'll appear more confident, and feel that way too. When you couple this change with the mental presence you developed in the previous chapter, you'll put yourself in the best possible position to dominate life.

To build a strong physical presence you must simply improve your posture. You must ensure that your body is a symbol of strength rather than weakness.

So, what is good, strong posture? It's most easily described by these 5 features:

1. The crown of the head is held high, as if someone were pulling your head towards the sky.

2. The shoulders are pulled back, as if you were trying to squeeze a nickel in between your shoulder blades. Regularly stretching your chest and doing back-dominant exercises like rows and pull ups will greatly assist you here.

3. You're not afraid to take up space, standing or sitting, to ensure your own comfort – picture a powerful mob boss sitting with one leg crossed, and both of his arms strewn out beside him.

4. You move with a slow and deliberate pace, and refrain from nervously jumping around or fidgeting.

5. You maintain strong eye contact, always holding it for slightly longer than your conversational partner. This demonstrates confidence, but side-steps the problem of scaring or intimidating those who struggle to maintain eye contact.

Adopt these 5 behaviors and take on the image, and the mentality, of a dominant leader. Do as Lenin did, and command respect with only the sight of your body.

CHAPTER 19

Chizuo Matsumoto was born in 1955 to a large, poor family in Japan. He was born with glaucoma and subsequently lost all sight in his left eye, and retained only partial vision in his right eye. This caused him to attend a school for the blind, and pursue a career in acupuncture – a traditional Japanese occupation for the blind.

His acupuncture education led him to studying Chinese fortune telling and meditation, and this eventually instilled a belief in him that he possessed supernatural powers. In 1984, Matsumoto changed his name to Shoko Asahara and started *Aum Shinrikyo*, a group that began as a simple meditation and yoga class in his one bedroom apartment.

Shoko quickly became more radical. In 1992, he declared himself to be "Christ" and preached a belief system that combined aspects of Christianity and yoga with the writings of Nostradamus. He promised his rapidly growing group of followers that he would take upon himself the sins of the world, and, in turn, absolve them of their sins and transfer to them a set of supernatural powers.

Over the next few years, the group continued to attract more members, and, at the same time, controversy and attention from the Japanese public. Leading up to 1995, Shoko and *Aum Shinrikyo* were involved in various murders of members who tried to leave, assassination attempts of heads of other religious sects, kidnappings, and weapons manufacturing.

In 1995, the group, now numbering as many as 9,000 followers in Japan and 40,000 worldwide, reached its boiling point. On March 20, Shoko ordered a number of the group's members to release sarin, a deadly nerve gas agent, onto five lines of the Tokyo subway. 13 people died, 50 were injured, and nearly 1000 temporarily went blind. He sits on death row in a Japanese prison cell to this day.

Rule 19: Speak in terms of their values and interests

Despite creating a violent cult, and using it for evil intentions, Shoko demonstrates a powerful concept that nearly all persuasive leaders throughout history took advantage of: speaking to other people in terms of their own interests.

The fact is that humans are inherently selfish. We care about our own lives and our own success. And this isn't a bad thing – we all need to take good care of our bodies and minds in order to prosper. But you must avoid the trap of becoming too self-centered and subsequently losing the ability to focus on other people.

Shoko gained his following by preaching something that was valuable to prospective members – forgiveness of sins and the promise of supernatural spiritual powers. Bear in mind, his prospective members were religious minded people with an inclination to believe controversial spiritual prophecies. He took advantage of this and gave them what they wanted – forgiveness and power.

When you deal with people, you must do the same. You must realize what it is that they want, and you must give it to them.

No, I don't mean that you should physically give them material gifts like money or cars. I also don't mean that you should offer them false promises to exploit them, like Shoko did. I used him as an example merely to demonstrate the power of this simple technique.

What I do mean is that you must be able to relate to the interests of whoever you're talking to. You must be able to identify and speak to what it is that motivates them. Doing this correctly will grant you instant influence and respect in their lives. It will allow you to open them up and operate on a far higher level than the man who simply drones on talking about his own problems and desires, both annoying and tiring his conversational partner. It will set you apart.

After you've built a strong mental and psychological foundation by believing that you'll succeed, and adopting the body language of a dominant individual, you must turn your attention outwards. Focusing your conversation on the other person is the final piece of the puzzle to creating an undeniable presence.

My Experience

I haven't started my own personal cult, but I have consciously used this principle many times. The freshest example in my mind is the last time I asked for a raise.

The single biggest mistake most guys make when asking for a raise is talking in terms of their own interests and accomplishment. On second thought, the biggest mistake guys make is not having the balls to ask for a raise in the first place. But when they do, they tend to fail miserably.

Put yourself in the shoes of an employer. If one of your workers comes to you and asks for more money, you sure as hell expect him to convince you that he's worth it. The last thing you want to hear is about how he's been working more hours or just had his biggest month in sales. Yes, these things please you, but in less he considering leaving immediately, it won't give you much reason to throw more of *your* money his way.

You must take the opposite approach and talk to your employer in terms of his interests. In my recent case, this meant telling him that if he increased my hourly rate by 33% I would be able to allocate more hours to his firm (as opposed to my other gigs). I continued to explain that this would translate to the ability for me to work on a large new project the company was just taking on, and I knew they were short-handed on. This would allow them to complete the project far sooner, and in a far more efficient manner.

He immediately saw the immense value I would bring to the table by granting me a raise, and promptly gave it to me – all because I spoke to him in terms of his interests, not my own.

Take Action

By focusing your conversations on other people and their interests, you're able to effectively use your mental confidence and strong physical presence to build influence, respect, and rapport in others. In short, it's the third wheel of the presence triangle that, when used together, will allow you assume the identity of socially dominant man.

To implement this principle into your life, simply start to approach all of your conversations with the purpose of speaking to your partner's interests. If you're asking for a raise, this means talking about what you can do for the company.

If you're trying to build rapport with a stranger, this is finding out what they like to do, and then asking them more about it. For example, anyone who talks to me about fitness or entrepreneurship immediately engrosses me into the conversation and quickly establishes themselves as a friend.

The applications for this concept are endless. If you're trying to build attraction with a girl you just met, you should push to learn facts about her, which you can in turn use to tease her. Most men make the deadly mistake of trying to talk themselves up or talk about things that they might have in common with the girl. Stop. She doesn't care about you yet. She cares about herself – use this to your advantage, make her feel comfortable in your presence, and then tease her and touch her to build attraction and make her feel dominated by your presence. Droning on about your *cool* job will only serve to bore her.

SUMMARY: A DOMINANT PHILOSOPHY

I'm confident that the advice inside this book can and will make you a dominant and accomplished man, who takes what he wants. If you learn from the successes of the powerful historical figures we've covered, and the experiences and mistakes that I've made, you'll be able to quickly adjust your course and make rapid progress towards getting to be exactly where – and who – you want to be.

I'll leave you with a brief review of each of the six major aspects of domination, and the related rules, so that you can begin to see the larger picture that's painted when everything is considered together in unison.

I. Death

The prospect of death is something that most men cower behind. They allow it to rule their lives, and keep them in check, hiding in a shady corner that leads nowhere.

You must do the opposite and **acknowledge your coming death**. You must embrace the inevitable so that you can free yourself from its chains. Do as the Tibetan Buddhist monks do, and perform the *Nine Point Meditation* to slowly condition yourself to accept your imminent demise.

Once you've begun to see the world through a more-accurate lens, you must use this as motivation to live your life fully and **value your time above all**. Realize that your time is your most precious commodity, as it can be used to accomplish or build anything you spend it on. Don't make the mistake of watching it wither away.

II. Fear

Similar to death, most men have become slaves to all of their fears: social fears, fears of failure, fears of poverty – the list goes on. They live their lives inside walls that their fears have built around them.

You must use a systematic approach to slowly and effectively free yourself from the powerful spell your fears hold over you. First, take the time to **identify your fears** by posing yourself the simple question: *what's holding me back from doing something that I want to do, or from exploring an opportunity that I'm interested in?*

Next, continue to hammer away at your fears by **understanding their causes**. Do this by asking yourself: *why's this holding me back from doing exactly what I want to?*

Once you understand the causes, you are in a much better position to take a chokehold on your life. But before you can move forward, you must first **determine the worst possible outcome** of facing a particular fear. This will remove any uncertainty and put you in a position of power from which you can dominate the fear.

The last step is to simply **confront your fear**. At the end of the day, this is the only step that will remove it from your life and allow you to live as you wish.

III. Direction

The cardinal sin the average man makes that keeps him average is failing to set goals for himself. A ship with no sail simply moves where the ocean takes it. You must set yourself apart, raise your sail, and take control of your life, and where it's headed.

Start by **creating a goal**. It doesn't matter exactly what it is – the simple fact that you have a mission will create a powerful sense of purpose in your life that will radiate from inside of you for the external world to see. Start with something small that you can achieve in a matter of weeks, to build momentum.

Next, **make a game plan** so that you're not throwing darts aimlessly in the dark. Most men fail to accomplish their goals because they don't make a game plan that grounds them in reality.

Finally, **embody the desired result** by taking on the persona of someone who's destined to accomplish his goal. Convince yourself of its inevitability by visualizing it being accomplished every day. This will put you in a class of your own, surrounded by the hopeless masses who struggle to start a diet or hit the gym.

And always be ready for obstacles to present themselves. They will test your grit and your determination. You must constantly be prepared to adjust your course and **persist until it's complete.**

IV. Action

Another common failing of the modern man is inaction. He prefers to sit there in the comfort of his own home and his own insecurities than actually start doing something different and ensuring that a direction that he chose for himself is actually realized.

The most common example of inaction is hesitation. **Don't hesitate**. Always act sooner rather than later, whether this means taking the first step of your game plan, or making a tough decision. Waiting will only lead to more waiting, and eventually you'll just give up and accept your lowly future.

Another way to take advantage of action is to actively monitor your life for new opportunities. When you fail to take advantage of new possibilities that are laid in front of you, you begin to take on the identity of someone who thinks he's *unlucky* – someone who believes that he can't catch a break. You must do the opposite and **make your own luck** by capitalizing on anything that's thrown your way – even by being creative and adapting seemingly unfavorable events to work in you favor.

Finally, you must **embrace the unknown**, because it's inevitable that you'll face opportunities where it's uncertain exactly what will happen if you choose to go forward. Rather than letting this paralyze you, accept that you won't move forward and get *lucky* if uncertainty rules your life. *Fortune favors the bold,* as they say.

V. Ownership

One of the biggest distinctions that can be made between a strong man and a weak man is their ability to take ownership of their actions. The weak man always chooses to pass the blame onto others. The strong man does not.

He **takes ownership of his successes and his failures**, realizing that passing the blame only serves to weaken his character, both in his mind and in the minds of those around him. He rises above the masses by always shouldering the burden of tough decisions and unfortunate circumstances.

Furthermore, he **doesn't allow the opinions of others to dictate his own self-worth**. He understands the inevitability of haters, both inside the camps of his enemies and his friends. Whereas the weak man lets criticism weigh him down and devalue his self-image, the strong man shakes it off and assumes complete ownership of his self-worth, remaining confident in the presence of insults and doubt.

Finally, he owns his life path and **creates his own identity**, rather than allowing himself to drift wherever life, or the expectations of others, takes him. He consciously chooses his next move, and then he executes it in spite of any opposition.

VI. Presence

The final part of dominating life and becoming the man you want to be is creating a powerful and confident social presence. You must be noticed before your even open your mouth – and you must command respect and develop influence afterwards.

The first step is to **establish a psychological foundation of success**. Use affirmations to fill your minds with thoughts of victory, and then proceed with the confidence and performance boost that this technique yields.

Next, you should **build a strong physical presence,** because people with good posture are always perceived as more confident. They also tend to take on a more confident mentality. So hold your head high, draw your shoulders back, take up space, and move with a deliberate pace.

There's one last step to ensure that you take advantage of the presence you've built. This is **always speaking to other people in terms of their values and interests**. Executing this principle will entice them to like you, listen to you, and respect you.

CAN YOU DO ME A FAVOR?

Thank you for buying and reading my book. I'm confident that you're well on your way to dominating life and becoming the man you want to be if you follow what's written inside.

Before you go, I have a small favor to ask. Would you take a minute to write a brief blurb about this book on Amazon? Reviews are the best way for independent authors (like me) to get noticed and sell more books. I also read every review and use the feedback to write future revisions – and future books, even.

Thank you.

MY OTHER BOOKS

If you enjoyed this book, you'll find my others awesome, too. They're all available on Amazon.

1. *The Book of Alpha: 30 Rules I Followed to Radically Enhance My Confidence, Charisma, Productivity, Success, and Life*

2. *Shredded Beast: Get lean. Build muscle. Be a man.*

3. *The Book of Bulking: Workouts, Groceries, and Meals for Building Muscle*

4. *The Simple Art of Bodybuilding: A Practical Guide to Training and Nutrition*

ABOUT THE AUTHOR

David De Las Morenas is an engineer, personal trainer, and internet entrepreneur known for his bestselling books on men's self-improvement and fitness. Follow him at **www.HowToBeast.com**, where he writes and shares more quality content.

www.ingramcontent.com/pod-product-compliance
Lightning Source LLC
Chambersburg PA
CBHW060406290526
45791CB00002B/633
* 9 7 8 1 4 9 7 5 1 8 1 6 2 *